DAY

Dr Dam
nutritio
and is a
Society fo

DAY LIGHT ROBBERY

Damien Downing

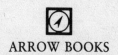

ARROW BOOKS

To my children,
Rachel and Marcus

Arrow Books Limited
62-65 Chandos Place, London WC2N 4NW

An imprint of Century Hutchinson Limited

London Melbourne Sydney Auckland
Johannesburg and agencies throughout
the world

First published 1988
Reprinted 1988

Phototypeset by Input Typesetting Ltd, London
Printed and bound in Great Britain
by The Guernsey Press Co. Ltd
Guernsey, Channel Islands

Contents

CHAPTER 1
Light starvation

The plot of many a thriller has hinged on the fact that the best place to hide something is where it is obvious. Our eyes are accustomed to noticing changes, movements and details, and rapidly come to ignore the things that we know are there and are unchanging. Our ears soon stop hearing the roar of traffic and focus on the conversation to which we want to listen. In dealing with health it is easy to see the immediate effects that a drug like aspirin has on pain and on temperature, but not so easy to appreciate the slow and subtle effects of diet on health. Indeed, it is little thanks to the medical profession that we are now becoming aware of dietary factors. Yet there is one factor so obvious, so all-pervading, that we appear to have missed it completely. That factor is sunlight.

The fact that we are now becoming aware of the enormous power of sunlight to improve our health is largely due to the life's work of one man – Dr John Ott. He is neither a scientist nor a doctor of medicine; perhaps this is why he lacked the blinkers of medical science and was able to see the obvious.

Throughout history, and particularly since the industrial revolution, man has been spending more and more of his time indoors. In other words, he has been progressively screening himself from the sunlight. Nowadays, it is possible to wake indoors, to travel to work in a car or train indoors, to work throughout the day indoors, to lunch and to return home by the same method to spend the hours of leisure indoors. Walking from car to work, and from work to lunch may be done between tall buildings where the sun hardly ever reaches. The only time when we see the sun is when we follow outdoor pursuits such as sport or gardening, or go on holiday. Is it only the strenuous exertion of sport which makes us feel better? Is it merely a coincidence that squash, which is a vigorous game played entirely indoors, has such a high risk of problems such as heart attacks associated with it? I shall describe how sunlight alone can have the same beneficial effect as exercise, and how the two of them together are even better.

Many degenerative diseases (heart disease, hardening of the arteries, blood pressure, pre-senile dementia, multiple sclerosis), as well as depression and other psychiatric problems, are much more common in Western society. Is this simply due to our poor diet, or is it also due to the fact that we live in temperate climates, with low levels of sunlight to begin with, and then spend most of our time indoors away from the sun?

And yet, you may say, we all know that sunlight causes skin cancer. This is not correct. Regular doses of sunlight appear to help in preventing most cancers. It is sun-burning, not sun-tanning, that may cause skin cancer. To live all year indoors and then to fry on holiday is comparable to taking all of one's yearly intake of alcohol in a fortnight. (Many people on the Costa Brava appear to be doing that too!)

An everyday problem

When I had read about the work of Dr Ott and other pioneers in this field, I started listening to my patients with an awareness of the possibility that light might influence their health. I tried not to lead them, or to encourage them to say anything about sunlight specifically, rather asking them about such things as the effect of the seasons on their health. I then heard a great many things which, if I had not been aware of the possibility of the sunlight effect, I would have been unable to hear.

Take as an example the case of Mrs A. In 1980 her periods stopped, and she started putting on weight. She gained three stones in two years. Then she developed pins and needles in her extremities, and had difficulty with walking. She was diagnosed as suffering from multiple sclerosis. When I asked her whether she could think of any events or changes in her lifestyle immediately preceding the start of her symptoms, she at first said no. A month later she told me that it had occurred to her that everything started when she began a new job, working in a modern health centre, in an entirely windowless room. She worked there until her symptoms became so bad that she had to stop work.

Take also Miss Y. When she came to see me she was twenty-two. Since the age of fourteen she had developed symptoms every year, at around Christmas-time, of lack of concentration, difficulty focusing, fuzzy-headedness, fatigue, generally feeling unwell, fluid retention and swelling, constipation, vomiting, purple discolouration of the extremities, a rash, and loss of the ability to taste and smell. These symptoms gradually worsened for two months, and then improved in the spring, clearing up by April. One year she spent a fortnight in the South of France in the autumn, and didn't become ill that winter. After this she found that she felt much better for having a course on a sunbed, but even better for having a holiday in the sun.

Both of these patients are made worse by lack of sunlight, and better by exposure to it. If we had not become aware of this fact, Mrs A. would have been diagnosed and treated as a case of multiple sclerosis, and Miss Y. would probably have been diagnosed as suffering from depression. How many thousands more people are suffering from lack of sunlight, without knowing it?

How many, indeed, know that January is their worst month, and try to arrange to spend it elsewhere than in this country? During the first two months of the year, the Canary Islands, our nearest winter hot spot, are full of people who know that they need a dose of sunlight.

Mr B. is a hairdresser; every winter, as well as feeling increasingly fatigued as the months went by, he developed a succession of colds and sore throats. He knew that the chemicals used in hairdressing (which may be the most toxic trade that exists in the 1980s) made his sore throat and all his other symptoms worse. But he also knew that he reacted more to them in winter than in summer. When I saw him in mid-January, he had already booked his week in Lanzarote, and was leaving the next day. 'It's the only thing that keeps me going in the winter,' he said.

Between 1900 and the start of World War II there were many scientific studies done on the benefits of sunlight. With the impetus provided by wartime needs, first antibiotics, then cortisone and steroids, then the major tranquillisers such as chlorpromazine were discovered. The drug industry was born. Today drug companies are among the largest of the great multi-nationals, and the vast bulk of medical research is oriented towards the effect of chemicals on disease. Sunlight has been forgotten.

In 1985 the three biggest selling antihypertensives (drugs to control blood pressure) had worldwide sales of 1.2 billion dollars.[1] Nobody was prescribed sunlight for their blood pressure, yet a single dose of sunlight can lower blood pressure for up to a week at no cost to the taxpayer. The higher your blood pressure, the greater the benefit you can derive from sunlight. No one has ever disproved the studies on the effect of sunlight that were done before the war. The medical community simply lost interest in them because of the more profitable effects of drugs. Subsequent chapters will discuss evidence that sunlight can help diseases ranging from athlete's foot and acne through heart disease and depression to senile dementia. It can improve hyperactivity, infertility, cancer, obesity, diabetes, bone fractures in old age, respiratory infections, and perhaps most pervasive of all, stress.

The man who started it all

In 1927 John Ott was a gangly, bespectacled teenager with poor health, which kept him off school quite often. This allowed him to develop his fascination with photography, and that year he photographed his first time-lapse sequence, of an apple blossom coming into flower. After two days of trying to dash back and forth, and setting his alarm clock at night to wake him up so that he could photograph the blossom every hour, he converted the old kitchen clock into an automatic timer. Now an elderly, respected researcher, he says that he keeps meaning to repair the kitchen clock, but it is still in use as a timer![2]

John Ott's fascination with time-lapse photography grew till he had a greenhouse and potting shed entirely devoted to growing plants and photographing them. He became a well-known TV personality in Chicago, with his Sunday afternoon botanical half-hour, and he made a number of films for Walt Disney. These are probably the best known of any time-lapse sequences in the world.

But there were a number of problems with getting the plants to grow when and how he wanted them to. Ears of corn, for instance, when grown in a glass greenhouse, were spindly and small. If he grew them outdoors they developed into normal healthy ears, but it is impossible to do time-lapse photography with a plant that is waving in the breeze. At this time, plastic sheeting was just coming on the market, and he found that his corn plants grew much better under plastic than under glass. It was only later that he realised the difference between them – plastic transmits ultraviolet light, but glass does not.

When growing flowers and plants in cold frames, it appears that nurserymen have always known that they would grow better if the glass was removed from the frame completely during the day. In fact, until World War II there was an ultraviolet-transmitting glass made in this country, largely for the greenhouse trade.

Light and colour

It was when he was attempting to film the flowering of a pumpkin for Walt Disney that John Ott came across the effect of colour on growth. Pumpkins can produce flowers of both sexes from one plant. But he found that if the pumpkin was grown under ordinary 'warm white' fluorescent light it produced male flowers which were healthy, but the female flowers withered. He then changed to a 'daylight' fluorescent light which provided a nearer approximation to visible daylight, and found that the male flowers withered but the female ones grew well.

If the plant was allowed to grow outdoors, of course, it naturally developed into a healthy, normal, bisexual pumpkin. But by this time things were getting desperate; he had spent two years unsuccessfully trying to film the life cycle of a pumpkin, he had only female flowers, and the season was drawing to a close.

He telephoned several friends in agricultural colleges and centres, but to no avail. He then tried further south, in Florida. The friend he called mentioned the problem to a reporter, and soon newspapers and TV across America were searching for a male pumpkin; the 'Cinderella pumpkin' was national news. Finally a lady in Florida called in to say that she had a male that was in flower. An airline offered to fly the plant straight up to Chicago, and Dr Ott rushed to the airport to collect his prize. The passengers were held up on the plane while 'Prince Pumpkin' was escorted off, to the popping of flash bulbs, and taken directly to his laboratory. In the nick of time, Dr Ott got his film sequence completed.

Another of Dr Ott's ambitious ventures was to build a complete mini-studio around an apple. He tells the story of this in his first book, *My Ivory Cellar*.[2] Looking rather like a birdwatcher's hide on wooden stilts, this had a glass window in the top, with shutters that would close to keep out the sun and protect the high-speed film necessary. It had three cameras, photographic lights, two thermostats and a fan. The tree itself was elaborately lashed so that it would not be moved by the wind.

The project went very well from March until late summer. Then all the other apples turned red and fell, but those inside the box remained green and continued to get bigger. Various gardening chemicals that were supposed to encourage fruit to ripen had no effect, and it was not until, in a subsequent year, he replaced the glass top with plastic that he finally managed to film a ripening apple turning red.

Fishes and men

Even a scientist could deduce from these results that light was a crucial factor in the development of plants. But Dr Ott was wiser than that; he speculated that the same might apply to animals. His next experiment was with fish eggs, and it proved him right. Using high intensity fluorescent lighting, and leaving it on for most of the twenty-four hours, he found that the fish stopped laying eggs entirely. It was only when the lights were restricted to eight hours every day that they started laying again. Then he found that the fish that were kept under pink fluorescent lighting produced almost entirely female offspring. In fact eighty per cent were females, and the remainder were of indeterminate sex.

The same effect was obtained with chinchillas and minks, and since then with a number of laboratory animals. It seems clear that the full spectrum of daylight is necessary for normal reproduction in mammals.

Dr Ott naturally then started to ask whether these effects might not apply to humans also. One of his earliest experiences in this direction was with his own health. He had worn glasses since childhood, and had been spending much of his life indoors under photographic lights. By middle age he was going bald, felt generally run down and suffered from frequent colds and respiratory infections, and had X-ray evidence of arthritis in his hip. This became so severe that he used a walking stick and an old bicycle to get from his house to the shed where the cameras were housed. Having heard that the Florida weather was reputed to be very beneficial to health, and that many people retired there for that reason, he spent a holiday on the beach there, sunbathing and relaxing, but experienced absolutely no benefit. During this time he always protected his eyes with sunglasses, or at least used his own spectacles.

Back in Chicago, and feeling no better, he happened to break his glasses. The spare pair were unwearable, so he was outside in the sun for several days without spectacles. All of a sudden, he noticed that he didn't seem to need the cane any more, and that his joints were generally much looser and easier. He walked cautiously up and down the drive, and then literally ran upstairs, for the first time in years, to tell his wife.

Deducing that sunlight was the factor, and that it was blocked by glasses, just as it had been blocked from the apple by the glass roof of the box, he went back to Florida for one week. During this time he never wore glasses, he tried to avoid driving in cars, and spent as much time as possible sitting out of doors in the shade. By the end of the week his arthritis had definitely improved, and he felt much fitter.

Thirty years later, Dr Ott is a fit, elderly gentleman who still lives in the town in Florida which he visited for that holiday. He continues his research, uses glasses only for small print, and even has a good head of grey hair. The regained years have not been wasted; Dr Ott has asked more piercing questions and stirred up more scientific controversy in his life than many of us can ever hope to read about.

He has established that exposing animals to daylight, or to full-spectrum lighting that closely mimics daylight, causes animals ranging from chickens to rabbits to produce more babies, and healthier ones too. As ever, he was quick to apply this finding to humans, and he now appears to have been successful in helping a number of couples with infertility, simply by telling them to sunbathe. Clearly this is the appropriate recommendation for Mrs A., whose periods stopped when she worked in an internal room. In Chapter 14 we shall see how sunlight stimulates the sexual hormones in both men and women.

Remarkably, Dr Ott also showed that when rabbits are reared in daylight rather than artificial light, their behaviour is much better. Usually, laboratory rabbits – and especially the males – are notoriously aggressive, even towards their own offspring. The males have to be separated from the litters, as they have a tendency to cannibalism. When they are reared under daylight, on the other hand, they are far from aggressive; the male rabbit actually helps to care for the litter, particularly when the mother is absent. He becomes a model parent. Serious food for thought in these days of child abuse.

Dr Ott showed that a strain of mice prone to fatal tumours lived twice as long on average in daylight as they did under pink fluorescent lighting. He later instigated a study of the effects of sunlight on cancer in humans – a study which was beginning to show exciting beneficial effects when it was suppressed by the medical establishment because they *knew* it couldn't be true. In Chapter 6 we shall discuss some new evidence that goes some way towards explaining how sunlight may help to cure cancer.

He also showed quite clearly that the radiation from a television screen was able to cause normal, healthy rats to become hyperactive and aggressive for about the first three to ten days, after which they became increasingly lethargic. This effect was screened out by the use of a lead sheet between the animals and the TV. Plants exposed in the same way behaved similarly; they grew rapidly at first, reaching abnormal heights, but then becoming unhealthy and deformed. These studies sparked off a national health investigation in the USA, which led to new regulations regarding the permissible levels of radiation from TVs.[3] We are only now starting to question the safety of televisions and VDUs, particularly for pregnant women.

Following on from these experiments he showed that artificial lighting could produce hyperactivity and disturbed behaviour in children – of which more later. Before World War II it was generally accepted, by the medical profession as much as by anyone, that sunlight was essential to the healthy development of children's bodies and minds. Parents were advised that exercise in the fresh air and sunlight were important, and children in hospital were taken out of doors in their cots to enjoy the sun. But nowadays we imagine that development will happen of its own accord and any problems can be dealt with by drugs. The critical parts played by sunlight and diet have been forgotten.

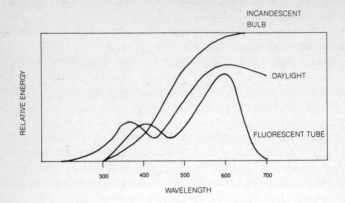

Full-spectrum lighting

Perhaps the most far-reaching of Dr John Ott's ideas is his invention of full-spectrum lighting. I believe that this may be the most important single public health measure of my lifetime.

From romantic candles to third-degree interrogations, lighting has always been used for its psychological impact. But we now appreciate that it can have an even greater physiological effect. Most of this comes from the invisible component of daylight and of full-spectrum lighting – the ultraviolet. Ordinary electric lights have a very limited spectrum of light, but full-spectrum lighting attempts to reproduce sunlight as closely as possible.

It does this either by using a fluorescent tube which has a wider spectrum of emission, reaching into the ultraviolet and taking in the blue end of visible on the way, or else – as in the most recent models, which Dr Ott now recommends – by combining a tube which produces all of the visible spectrum with a small ultraviolet tube. Most full-spectrum lights now have devices to block other potentially toxic radiations which might leak out.

Throughout more than half a century of pioneering research,

Dr Ott has clearly demonstrated that full-spectrum lighting is beneficial. He has instigated or participated in many research projects on the health effects of light, and has published several books. He has been rewarded with a number of honorary doctorates and other academic awards. But he makes no pretence of being a scientist; if he were, he might not have had the vision and courage to ask the questions that he did.

Degrees and doctorates notwithstanding, his greatest reward has to be the gratitude of untold numbers of people, now and in the future, who will be helped by his ideas. Without his genius, this book would never have been imagined, still less written. I believe that his ideas, and the discoveries and inventions they have led to, will change the way we live – and to save and improve millions of lives.

CHAPTER 2
The entropy machine

Do you remember entropy? If you did physics at school, you probably will; if not, never mind, because it is a surprisingly simple concept once you get the hang of it. The second law of thermodynamics states that the energy in a system always tends to degenerate from order into chaos. The most obvious example is that heat dissipates. If you leave a hot cup of tea standing for half an hour, most of the heat in it will have been lost. The heat energy in the tea has spread outwards into the area around it – the cup, the table it was standing on, and the air surrounding it.

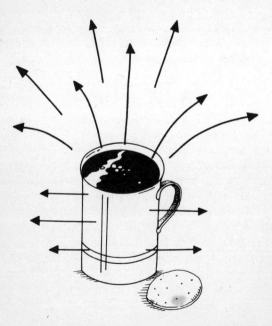

You started with heat energy that was useful because it was all contained in a small object that you could utilise – the cup of tea. When this heat energy became spread more thinly throughout the room, it was of no further use to you. Entropy describes this process of heat loss, but it also describes a general rule that energy of any kind is eventually lost and wasted, spread into the rest of the universe. Mostly, it ends up as heat energy which diffuses outwards – just like that in the cup of tea.

The green net

On earth, all energy, whether stored in living organisms, in machines, in the weather or the potential energy of water in high places, originates from the sun and gradually gets degraded into heat energy which diffuses outwards to equilibrate with heat around it, and is lost into space. This is entropy. All life is a system for trapping energy, and thereby for defying entropy. Entropy is the supreme antilife force of the universe, the downward slope from the pure energy of sunlight to the empty wastes of outer space. This is the slope on which we live our lives, and down which we struggle not to slide. To this end there is a certain amount of teamwork between the different organisms on our planet.

The biggest and best energy trap in the world is photosynthesis in green plants. The leaves of such plants have an array of structures called 'light-harvesting antennae'. Each of these consists of around three hundred molecules of chlorophyll, the pigment which gives plants their green colour, surrounding a single 'reaction centre'. As we shall later be looking at the importance of the mineral magnesium to human health, it is worth noting here that at the heart of the chlorophyll molecule sits an atom of magnesium, which gives it its shape and therefore its function.

The energy of sunlight is absorbed by the 'antennae' of chlorophyll molecules, and transmitted, rather like a chain of dominoes falling, from molecule to molecule inwards to the reaction centre.[1] Here there is a complex system of enzymes which uses the energy supplied to it by the chlorophyll to combine the carbon dioxide and water into carbohydrates. In the process oxygen is released into the atmosphere.

$$CO_2 + H_2O \rightarrow (CH_2O) + O_2$$

These carbohydrates are the prime source of energy for life on this planet; not just for plants but also for animals and humans. In our bodies a complex biochemical cycle called the Krebs cycle breaks down the molecules of carbohydrate in our food, step by step, into carbon dioxide and water again, extracting the stored energy at each stage and sending it off in biochemical form to be used throughout our bodies. The carbon dioxide is breathed out into the atmosphere, where it can be used again by plants in photosynthesis.

$$(CH_2O) + O_2 \rightarrow CO_2 + H_2O$$

Although photosynthesis wastes a vast majority of the energy available to it, having an estimated efficiency of only 0.2 per cent (it wastes 99.8 per cent of the energy it receives), it is still the major energy trap for all life on our planet.[2]

Similarly, plants take up atoms such as carbon and nitrogen, and 'fix' them into their tissues. We eat the plants and utilise the proteins and other molecules that contain the carbon and nitrogen. When we excrete and when we die, these elements return to the soil, where they can again be used by plants. We are only one part of a cycle, the wheel of life, which needs to balance in order to keep going round. The destruction of the forests of the world to make paper and provide wood for building disturbs the balance by reducing the amount of oxygen available for us to breathe and increasing the carbon dioxide in the atmosphere.

Over the millennia, plants and animals have developed some ingenious mechanisms for coexistence, with animals depending on photosynthesis in plants for their food sources, and plants depending on animals, from pollinating bees to agricultural man, for the survival of their species. But photosynthesis predates animals by millions of years, so it clearly did not develop for

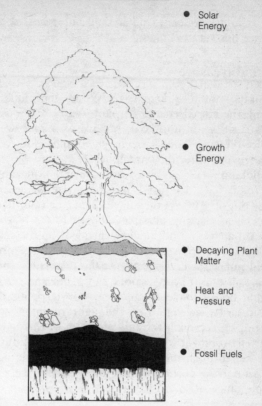

Solar
Energy

Growth
Energy

Decaying Plant
Matter

Heat and
Pressure

Fossil Fuels

the purpose of feeding them. We of the animal kingdom are, in
a sense, parasites on the plant world; we survive by being more
adaptable or more sophisticated or clever than plants, and we
have developed a variety of other mechanisms for trapping and
using the sun's energy.

These include the synthesis of vitamin D in the skin to improve
our absorption of minerals; the triggering of certain enzymes
that repair our DNA; the activation of oils on our skin by
sunlight to make them antiseptic and protective; the production
of hormones in the skin, in response to sunlight, that stimulate

our immune systems, and a range of other mechanisms that science has yet to explain.

Buried treasure

Mankind has also invented his own ingenious methods for taking the stored energy of photosynthesis by using the fossil fuels such as oil and coal, but we as a race were alive long before these methods were invented and, God willing, we will be alive long after they are gone.

Looking at the graph of fuel consumption you will see that the fossil fuels are just a passing phase we will be forced to grow out of. And yet they have changed all our lives drastically. As well as making possible modern forms of transport, they mean that we are no longer dependent on the sun for warmth or light, and so we can live in places where previously man could not survive. They also make it possible for us to spend nearly all of our time indoors, out of the sun.

Our bodies have mechanisms for trapping the energy in particular wavelengths of the light reaching earth, and we depend on receiving the full spectrum of this light. This is the light environment for which we are designed. But indoor light, whether through the windows or from electric lights, provides only a narrow portion of this full spectrum. Take a look at the whole range of solar radiation.

The light programme

All of these wavelengths are produced all the time by the colossal nuclear reactor that makes up the sun. If we could hear electromagnetic waves, they would sound like the 'white noise' that you get between stations on a radio or TV. But most of these wavelengths were filtered out by the earth's atmosphere, and only a narrow waveband arrives at ground level. This waveband stretches from the ultraviolet to the infra-red, with visible light making up the middle part of the spectrum. Solar radiation at ground level can therefore be divided into three components:

Past and projected world consumption of oil and coal

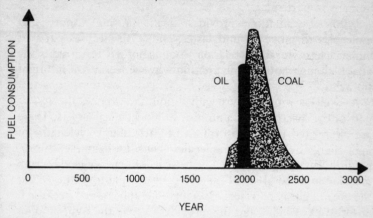

Figure 3

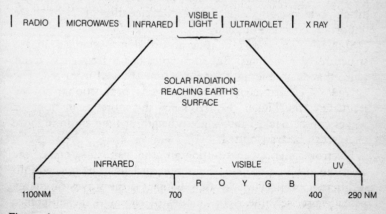

Figure 4

infra-red, visible and ultraviolet. Each of the three components of sunlight has particular effects on organisms in general, and humans in particular.

Infra-red radiation provides heat, causing atoms and molecules to move around faster, and it also causes parts of molecules to vibrate in relation to one another. Infra-red is the major, though not the only, reason why we feel warm in bright sunlight.

As well as providing us with vision and colour, the *visible* part of the spectrum has a number of biochemical effects. These are all related to the absorption of particular wavelengths of light energy by particular molecules. Thus, for example, chlorophyll in leaves appears green because it uses energy chiefly from the blue and red areas of the spectrum for photosynthesis, but the green light is reflected. Haemoglobin appears red because it absorbs green light, and this provides exactly the right amount of energy to shift a molecule from one structure or state to another. In other words, the light energy is absorbed by the molecule and converted into structural energy. The biochemical effects of the visible spectrum are much better researched in plants and bacteria than in man, but there is some very interesting evidence that particular wavelengths of light have important effects on humans.

Similarly, *ultraviolet* light is absorbed into changes in the structure of molecules. But ultraviolet has a frequency about twice that of visible light, or three times that of infra-red. The energy of electromagnetic radiations is proportional to the frequency; the higher the frequency the more oscillations or waves can be packed into a given length or time, and the more energy can be transmitted.

Electromagnetic waves hitting an atom can cause one of the electrons orbiting around the atomic nucleus to be pushed into a different orbit. This can only happen if the waves of energy provide precisely the right amount of energy – the difference between the atom's energy level at one orbit and at the other. If the energy provided is insufficient the electron will fall back to its original orbit, and if it is too great it may fly off into obscurity.

When an electron returns to a lower energy state, a lower orbit around an atom, it gives off electromagnetic radiation, the wavelength of which is determined by the amount of energy provided, which in turn depends on the difference in energy between the two orbits. This two-way process is crucial to the whole of life. It has also made possible much of modern biochemistry, because by measuring the wavelengths of radiation that are absorbed or emitted, we can calculate the energy changes that have occurred.

For example, one of the most basic techniques in the biochemistry laboratory is called spectrophotometry (wavelength-light-measuring). This involves selecting a particular wavelength of light, usually in the ultraviolet, and measuring the amount of light of that wavelength that a chemical emits or absorbs. The more of the chemical there is, the more light it sends out or soaks up. This is not a way of getting around nature – it is using the very basis of life as a measuring stick.

Everywhere in the world, around us and within us, living cells are sending and receiving signals in the form of light. But it took the genius of Albert Einstein to realise, and to demonstrate, that light and matter are interchangeable – that $E=mc^2$. Light is not just a pleasant side-effect of summer; the whole world runs on light energy.

CHAPTER 3
Skin tones and sun zones

Man's original home address is the Olduvai Gorge, East Africa.
To the best of contemporary archaelogical knowledge, that is
where we emerged as a species. From there, over the past four
million years, we have spread out to cover the whole land mass
of the planet. We cannot tell what colour of skin the original
hominids had, or how much hair, but everybody who is
indigenous to East Africa and other tropical countries nowadays
has very dark skin. The tribes that have spread north and south
have progressively lighter skin the further they live from the
equator.

The only obvious value of this difference in terms of survival
is that white skin transmits more light than dark skin. In general,
the further you are from the equator, the less sunlight there is
available. In fact, as the diagram shows, nearly everywhere

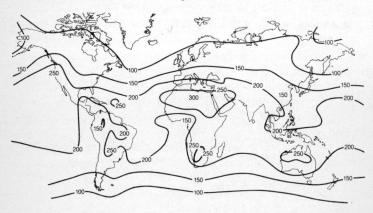

Exposure to light during a normal day

on or near the equator gets twice as much sunlight as Great Britain, and East Africa gets nearly three times as much.

In this respect, at least, we are adapted to the solar environment in that part of the planet in which we live. But from the beginning of history, and particularly since the atrocities of the slave trade, men have moved or been moved in large numbers from one part of the world to another. Nowadays, many of us are black people living in temperate climates, or white people living in the tropics. There are fair-skinned people of Celtic origin living in Queensland, Australia, one of the hottest and sunniest places on earth, for example, and people from the Indian subcontinent living in Birmingham. The former get skin problems from overdoses of sunlight, although there appears to be more to this story than a simple overdose effect; the latter get rickets due to vitamin D deficiency, even though they live on a diet which prevented rickets when they were in their home countries. For these reasons alone, sunlight must be regarded as a major health factor – but there is more.

Melanin

The chemical which produces darkness of skin and protects us from damage from sunlight is called melanin. The amino-acid tyrosine, which we get from our diet, is converted in our bodies by an enzyme to dopa. Sunlight activates an enzyme in the skin which produces a polymer of dopa (a polymer is a large molecule consisting of a chain of small molecules all the same.) This polymer is melanin. In people who are genetically dark-skinned the activity of this enzyme is high throughout life, so they always have more melanin. The same molecule gives black colouration to hair.

People who are genetically light-skinned, particularly Celts with red hair and freckles, produce little or no melanin. Instead they produce a different polymer, made up of another amino-acid, called cysteine, which imparts a red colour to hair. These people only ever tan to a very slight degree, and are therefore much more vulnerable to sun-burning. This is known as Type

One skin. In everybody else sunlight stimulates the tyrosinase enzyme to produce more melanin.

There are two phases to this; within the first hour of exposure to sunlight, there is a rapid production of a small quantity of melanin (this is known as IPD, or immediate pigment darkening). Over the next few days there is a slower production of a larger quantity, known as melanogenesis, which provides the major sun-tanning effect. Sun-burning, when the skin becomes red and tender, is a sign of damage to the skin by sunlight, and is not necessary for sun-tanning.

Skin types

It is possible to divide the world's people into six different skin types, according to their colouration and response to sunlight. The importance of this is not how much sunlight we need – we all need sunlight and benefit from it – but in just how much we can get away with.

If you are born with Type One skin, it is clearly not a very wise move to live in Ethiopia or the Arizona Desert, but if you have Type Five or Type Six skin then it may be equally bad for you to live in temperate climates, because your high skin melanin content will increase the effect of climate in filtering out ultraviolet light, and may cause you a light deficiency.

It is equally clear that if you have lived for months in a light-poor environment, to switch to spending much of the day undressed in a light-rich environment, as so many of us do on our annual holiday, is bound to be more than a pale skin can quickly adapt to. This much has been said over and over again by journalists in women's magazines and elsewhere; but unfortunately the overall effect has often been to lead us to believe that sunlight is bad for us in any amount and in any form. Such an idea goes counter to common sense, as well as to the cumulative body of scientific knowledge.

It is simply a matter of dosage. Just as our body requires carbohydrate to produce energy in order to function properly, but will suffer overdose effects if fed too much, so we require

SKIN	OCCURRENCE	APPEARANCE	SENSITIVITY TO SUN
1	Celtic	White skin, freckles, blue eyes red or blond hair	Burn very easily Do not tan
2	Northern Races	White skin, with/without freckles blue or hazel eyes, red or blond hair	Burn easily Tan slowly and slightly
3	Most white people	Fair skin, blond or brunette	Brown moderately Tan slowly and moderately
4	Mediterranean, Chinese, Japanese, Red Indian	Olive or light brown skin, dark hair, dark eyes	Burn slightly Tan easily
5	Indians, Arabs, Malaysians, Mexicans	Brown skin, hair and eyes brown or black	Burn rarely Tan well and deeply
6	Negroes, Aborigines	Skin brown to black, hair and eyes black	Never burn Remain dark-skinned

sunlight to stay healthy, but can suffer from an overdose if we are careless or stupid. Unfortunately, in our Western society, overdoses of carbohydrates are more common than underdoses; but a deficiency of sunlight is the general rule, and an overdose is hard to come by without travelling hundreds of miles to much hotter countries.

Light deficiency

The problem is made much worse by electricity. Lighting and heating run on electric power enable us to stay indoors for as long as we wish. In prehistoric times, whether we lived in East Africa or West Sussex, we had to spend much of the daylight hours out of doors. Many societies in the Third World still do, and for the same reasons. Firstly, in a non-technological agricultural society everybody's muscle power is needed for the work of raising food. Secondly, the lack of adequate indoor lighting means that most things that involve vision have to be done out of doors – or at least by an open window.

Nowadays we spend around ninety per cent of our time indoors – in offices, schools and homes – where the light level

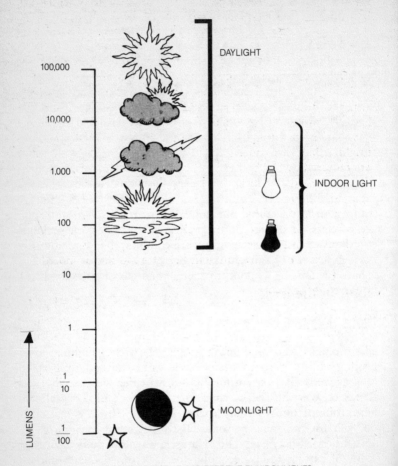

INTENSITY OF LIGHT IN DIFFERENT ENVIRONMENTS

is usually around one hundredth of that of midday sunlight.[1] Because our eyes adapt well and rapidly, better than any automatic camera, we are unaware of the difference after the first few seconds.

The illustration uses a logarithmic scale, so that the brightness of bright noonday sunlight is about one thousand times that of twilight. The official guidelines for indoor illumination set the required brightness level at somewhere between two hundred and one thousand lux.[2] This is around twilight level. Midday sunlight, even through cloud, should be more than ten times brighter than this. Indeed, it is daylight sunshine intensities that are required by our bodies for a number of functions, including the suppression of melatonin from the pineal gland, which is discussed in the next chapter. This requires a minimum intensity of 2500 lux, compared to the probably maximum of 1000 lux in indoor office environments.[3] Certain body functions, such as the regulation of human sleep-wake cycles and other biorhythms, require exposure to intensities of 4000 lux or more.

Kept in the dark

When scientists attached light detectors to the wrists and head of volunteers for stretches of a day or more, they found that their subjects were only infrequently exposed to anything over 1000 lux. They appeared to spend most of their time at an average intensity of around 100 lux. Yet this study was conducted in San Diego, which is one of the sunniest places in the continental USA.[4]

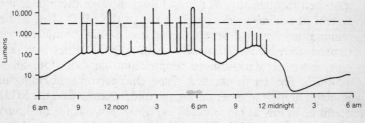

Light exposure throughout the 24 hours

According to the evidence now to hand, we clearly need considerably more sunlight than we receive. We need both a greater intensity of light, and for a longer period. To give an example, light of the intensity that is normally experienced in offices and other indoor environments is only half as effective in shifting human biorhythms backwards or forwards as a weak electrical AC field (of 10 hertz, and 2.5 V/m). This electrical field cannot be perceived consciously.[5]

When the light intensity rises above 2500 or 3000 lux, on the other hand, there is a major difference. It becomes possible to produce distinct effects on human metabolism and diurnal rhythms. Shift workers and transatlantic travellers should pay attention; bright light for three hours per day can retrain your wake/sleep cycle in forty eight hours.[6] Doing it with alarm clocks and coffee can take up to eight days.

The light frequency most effective at suppressing melatonin and therefore at altering biorhythms is between 450 and 550 nanometres.[7] This is blue and green light. The effect spills over into the ultraviolet, but there is virtually no effect from the higher — yellow and red — frequencies. The level of light that is required for melatonin suppression is roughly that of a cloudy day. It does not require blinding summer sunlight, but the light available under dark storm clouds is likely to be insufficient, as is indoor lighting.

Good medicine

For all the other benefits of sunlight which appear to be mediated through the skin rather than through the blood, the system of scaling works on the basis of the MED. This is the minimal erythemal dose: the amount of sunlight required just to produce reddening of the skin. Naturally this varies with skin type, extremely dark-skinned people requiring about four times as much. For a pale-skinned, Type One person sunbathing in England in high summer during the middle of the day, the MED might be as low as ten minutes' exposure. But outside the hours of 10 a.m. to 2 p.m., and outside the summer months of June,

July and August, it may be impossible for even a Celtic skin to achieve the MED.[8]

In any case, it is not advisable to do so. The MED is only useful as a reference point. Several Russian studies have shown that the ideal starting level for regular therapeutic solar exposure is around half of the MED (0.3 to 0.6 MED).[9] As the skin becomes accustomed to the exposure, this can be built up to as much as 1.5 times the original MED.

Using sunlight as therapy is clearly far easier in hotter countries and those with more predictable weather than Great Britain. In order to avoid light deficiency, most UK residents will need either to travel abroad regularly, or to use artificial lights. The concept of full-spectrum lighting, developed by John Ott, is an attempt to provide a reasonable replication of the frequency pattern of sunlight. There are a number of technical problems involved. For example, nearly all plastic and glass diffusers used to house fluorescent lighting will absorb effectively all of the UV. There is no point, therefore, in putting full-spectrum lights inside them. Some modern light housings, however, have metallic-coasted grid diffusers, with no glass or plastic obstructing the light path.

Using such lighting, aimed directly at the face from a short distance, it would be possible for some Type One individuals to develop an erythema after a day's exposure. Since this would be uncomfortably hot and likely also to produce a headache, no matter what form of lighting was used, few people would want to adopt it as a policy. Under normal indoor lighting levels, skin reddening only occurs as a result of other exposures, such as the ionisation from computer screens.

Therefore, we keep ourselves for most of our lives in perpetual twilight. All our images of freedom – and many of those used by advertisers to portray health – involve being out of doors and in the country. Locking people up in dungeons and prisons has always been a major form of punishment. Depriving man of the light is nearly as bad as depriving him of his life. Yet nowadays we live, without realising it, in self-imposed dungeons. Man is born to the light, and is everywhere in the dark.

CHAPTER 4

If you lived in Tibet you'd need three eyes

The health consequences of sunlight, and of light deprivation, have been appreciated intuitively since the dawn of man, but modern science is now making it possible to understand some of the mechanisms involved. One of the most important, and most obvious, is the effect of light on our cycle of waking and sleeping. This is chiefly mediated through a molecule called melatonin, which is produced by the pineal gland.

The pineal has often been referred to by mystical teachers, particularly from the East, as the third eye. The implication is that it perceives something above the awareness of our normal brain power. We now know the major 'cosmic' factor it responds to is light. Melatonin production only occurs in the pineal, in darkness, at night; and it sends us to sleep.[1]

Circadian rhythms

Until the arrival of the electric light there was a natural rhythm to our lives. In the daytime, sunlight made it possible for us to go out, to work and to travel. It was a time for expending our energy in the natural purpose of life. At night we retired indoors to the warmth of our cave or house, did very little and slept. This is the first and most basic biorhythm, and one that we share with all mammals.

Nowadays we still have the same bodies and the same biorhythms, but we ask of them that they be active at strange times of the day and night. Many nurses, factory workers and others have to work permanent nights, and many more of us have to work shifts. Ask anybody who works this kind of schedule what their body tells them; do they feel that it is good for them? We have abolished night, yet we have deprived ourselves of the sun.

Now that it is possible to get anywhere in the world in about twenty four hours by jet, many of us regularly cross time zones and suffer jet lag as a consequence. Although a significant component of jet lag is dehydration caused by the high altitudes, and indeed there may be other symptoms from the atrocious food that many airlines serve, it is clear that the major component is a disturbance of the day/night biorhythm. A flight from New York to London, or vice versa, results in a shift of five time zones. Therefore, what was bedtime becomes either the middle of the night or the middle of the afternoon. We either wake up in the small hours and fall asleep at our desk in the afternoon, or the other way round. In fact, many people find that the adrenalin of travel keeps them going for twenty four to forty eight hours after arrival, but then it hits them with a vengeance. Under normal circumstances it takes at least five days to adjust your biorhythm to the new time zone, and the unaccustomed waves of fatigue or attacks of insomnia may linger for up to a fortnight.

Interestingly, when humans are allowed to adjust their own wake/sleep cycles in an environment which gives no clues at all as to time, they invariable select a cycle that is significantly longer than twenty four hours. Results have varied between twenty five and twenty eight hours.[1] Ageing hippies may recall that Imanuel Velikovsky used this as an argument for his theory that the earth's rotational cycle had been altered by the impact of a giant comet, which also caused Noah's flood.[2] Such speculations aside, this internal rhythm explains why the short changeover on a shift system is always more gruelling. When

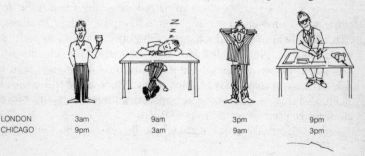

| LONDON | 3am | 9am | 3pm | 9pm |
| CHICAGO | 9pm | 3am | 9am | 3pm |

the time zone change requires that we turn our watches forward, this reduction in the length of a day goes counter to our natural tendency to a cycle slightly longer than twenty four hours.

The body's light meter

Tryptophan is an amino-acid that occurs naturally in our food. It is known to have a sedating effect. In fact the very high concentrations of tryptophan in meat are thought to explain why lions go to sleep after feeding on a kill, dozing in the sun for anything up to three days before they get hungry again. Tryptophan also makes us feel full. Tryptophan is very good at crossing the blood-brain barrier. This is the filtering of the bloodstream, only allowing certain chemicals across into the cerebrospinal fluid which bathes the brain.

As it crosses into the brain, tryptophan appears to carry a lot of amino-acids with it, effectively nourishing the brain. But its most important results are inside the brain, where it appears to relax and sedate. Yet tryptophan has no direct sedative action itself; it has to be converted to serotonin to achieve this. And serotonin is converted by the pineal into melatonin. Here at last it seems that we may have found the real natural sedative.

When melatonin was given to volunteers in scientific studies, it had effects very similar to those of a sleeping tablet. That is, it made them more sleepy, reduced their energy levels and reduced their performance on tests of motor function. Their reaction times on straightforward tests became longer, although they did not make any more mistakes.[3] The memory of the subjects in this test was not impaired at all by melatonin, in contrast to the effect of the benzodiazepine drugs (Valium, Ativan, Librium etc) which are commonly used as hypnotics and relaxants. Nevertheless, some of the melatonin subjects did fall asleep in the middle of the day. Given as a tablet, it seems that melatonin might have some potential as a tranquillisers and sleeping tablet – and some serious advantages over the more commonly used drugs now available.

Other effects of melatonin include increasing the sensitivity of subjects to barbiturates and other hypnotic drugs, enabling them to send the subjects to sleep even more quickly. It reduced the subjects' sensitivity to painful stimuli such as heat,[4] so they took longer to respond. It also appears to lower blood sugar, and to increase the activation (conversion into the active form) of pyridoxine, vitamin B6.[5] This vitamin is known to have a degree of anti-anxiety effect, as well as being important in the regulation of dreaming. According to Carl Pfeiffer, individuals who are deficient in B6 do not recall their dreams. When adequate B6 is administered, they have pleasant dreams, in colour, which they recall the following day.[6]

In other words, melatonin is produced by the pineal at times of darkness not only to stop us from being wakeful and doing things, but to prepare us for sleep as well. Because sleep is important as a time for wound healing and repair of tissues – and of injuries to the mind also, even though they may only be cuts and grazes. Whatever powerful spiritual and psychological functions sleep may have, its most basic mental function is to allow the mind to sort out the confusion of the day, throwing away the dross and filing the useful items. Melatonin potentiates all of this.

Regulating the pineal

The only way of synchronising bodily rhythms to a new time zone is by controlling melatonin levels – either by taking it orally or by adjusting the pineal's rhythm of output. Giving melatonin orally brings on sleep at the desired time; the draw-back of this, of course, is that there is no corresponding signal for turning off melatonin production, but it does appear to be effective in shifting our wake/sleep rhythm.[7]

It is also possible to influence the melatonin production of the pineal by electromagnetism. Artificial magnetic fields of a similar strength to the natural magnetic field of the earth can inhibit melatonin synthesis.[8] The effect depends on the intensity and the rhythm of the fields, but this finding ties in with other studies which have shown that such fields can affect the production of steroids by the adrenal, the movement of calcium into and out of cells, and even the synthesis of DNA in chromosomes. It has been suggested that disturbances of the geomagnetic field are related to mental and physical illnesses and death.[9] Some researchers have speculated that the changes in geomagnetic fields on a diurnal cycle and on an annual cycle may be important in adjusting melatonin rhythms. This research has a long way to go, however, and does not alter the fact that the strongest effect known on the pineal is produced by bright light entering the eye.

When we are exposed to bright light entering our eyes, our pineals stop producing melatonin within about half an hour. This can even be done in the middle of the night, when our melatonin production is naturally at its highest. But it works best in the morning, when our bodies are prepared for it. So while melatonin is nature's sleeping draught, our natural wake-up medicine is sunlight. Who needs coffee when the real thing is available for free? Personally I've become hooked on stepping outside first thing in the morning, and may often be seen walking the dog at 6.30 a.m., unshaven and carrying a mug of herb tea.

We know that it's not simply a psychological response, though, because it can still happen in blind people.[10] However, it is abolished with loss of the eyes themselves. This is because the pathway starts with the reception of light by cells in the retina but then travels by a different set of nerves from the optic nerve, which carries visual signals. This pathway leads by a circuitous route to the pineal, where the signal is given to turn off melatonin synthesis. In other words, our bodies give us a nightly dose of internal hypnotics, thereby keeping us in phase with the outside world and ensuring that we get the rest and recovery time provided by sleep. Because of its lack of side effects (no confusion or loss of memory, no addiction) melatonin would have great potential as a more natural sleeping tablet, and no doubt any drug company that could produce it would do a service both to mankind and to its investors. But we can produce our own melatonin without chemical assistance, if we understand how it is produced, and how that production is inhibited.

Although light entering the eye inhibits melatonin production, there are two obvious limiting factors on this. The first is that the most effective light is between about 460 and 560 nanometres in wavelength, which is blue and green light.[11] Red and yellow light has no effect at all, but there is an effect, it seems, in the ultraviolet.

This coincides with the peak intensity of natural sunlight, but unfortunately ordinary incandescent light bulbs produce much less at this wavelength than at the red end of the spectrum. Fluorescent lights produce more blue, which is why they tend to look whiter than incandescent bulbs, but they tend to have a trough of intensity right in the middle of the melatonin suppression range. Neither of them produce any ultraviolet at all. Therefore indoor lighting is bound to be poor at suppressing melatonin.

The second problem is that a minimum brightness of about 2500 lux is required to suppress melatonin, and indoor lighting rarely, if ever, reaches this intensity. So there is little chance of indoor light being useful in controlling melatonin, and thus our wake/sleep rhythm. The importance of this on a worldwide scale is impossible to estimate, but we do know that millions suffer transient sleep disturbances, as well as drowsiness and fatigue during the day. These may be due to physical illness, or simply a response to the stresses of life. Whatever the cause, if we can get a good night's sleep, and stay alert through the day, it is bound to be a help.

Disturbances of the wake/sleep cycle are also a recognised feature of the affective disorders – depression, anxiety and manic-depressive illness. Since 1983 there have been several studies which have shown that a dose of 'bright' light, of a mimimum intensity of 1500 lux (which means that is likely to have been borderline in effect), for a period of only one hour, can produce a significant but small improvement in mood as well as in sleep, in all types of depressed patients.[12] The effect was not limited to any one type of depression. The obvious comment on this is that a longer period of brighter light might well be even more beneficial. If you think it might help you, try it; there's nothing to lose.

Bodily depression

The medical model of depression says that it is a distinct illness which calls for specific treatment. One of the major pointers to a diagnosis of depression is a disturbance of sleep pattern. However, any doctor in clinical practice who takes the time to talk to his patients about this will confirm that large numbers of people with all kinds of illnesses complain, among other things, of minor variations in mood, of fatigue and lack of energy, and of disturbances of their sleep cycle. How many of these might feel better if they established their natural daily biorhythm again, using sunlight or bright indoor light which mimics sunlight?

Sad cases

There is a small group of people with depression who have a clear worsening in winter, and this is known as SAD – seasonal affective disorder. The characteristics of this are rather different from ordinary depression. The large majority of patients appear to swing the other way in summer months, to some extent, and their symptoms when they are depressed are rather different. Two thirds of them admit to a carbohydrate craving and to an increase in weight, as well as disturbances of the menstrual cycle. Interestingly, the disease usually starts earlier than ordinary depression with an average onset age of twenty two, and seventy per cent of them admit to at least one relative with a major depression or other affective disorder.[13]

These people feel better when they are nearer the equator, and they almost invariably improve when treated with bright light, of over 2500 lux. They get worse again when given mela-tonin capsules; as well as the usual drowsiness and slowing down, they develop much the same depressive symptoms as they experience in the depths of winter.

In the spring

In other words they are more sensitive to variations in the sunlight cycle than the rest of us. This does not mean that they are unique, or that the rest of us are free of such effects. There are at least forty variables that have been shown to have a seasonal difference, ranging from growth rates in children through sensitivity to dental pain to the alertness of train drivers.[14] The variation in growth rate was first described in 1886. The fascinating thing about all the studies on growth is that they show a completely opposite phase for increases in height and increases in weight. Children in a number of temperate climates grow most in height in late spring and early summer, just at the time when their weight gain is at its lowest. There can be as much as a fifty per cent difference between summer and winter in the rate of growth, and up to one hundred per cent range for weight gain.

Excretion of hormones in the urine varies by a similar degree. The principal male hormone, testosterone, is known to be produced by the effect of sunlight on the skin, and particularly on the skin of the genitals.[15] It is not surprising, therefore, that its levels rise throughout the spring and summer months, being about one third higher by the end of August than in February. Little wonder, too, that the peak month for conceiving babies is June. In the spring, a young man's fancy evidently does turn to thoughts of love – and by summer he's done something about it.

The levels of 17-ketosteroids, the adrenal steroids, which are produced in response to stress, on the other hand, fall steadily to a trough in August. The further north of the equator, the more marked is the trend. Clearly, at these latitudes our bodies find winter something of a strain.

The big sleep

Death from all causes peaks in January. This is hardly news, and does not have to be attributed to a direct effect of sunlight.

PLASMA TESTOSTERONE LEVEL

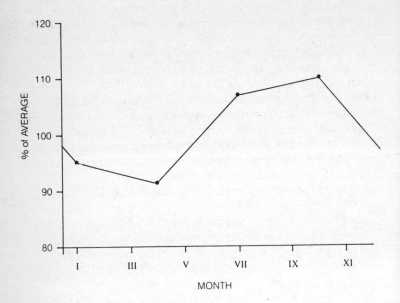

Some of the reasons are obvious. Respiratory infections, for instance, are more common in winter, as any GP will confirm. This is probably connected with the poorer supply of fresh vegetables leading to lower levels of vitamins, causing us to have weaker immune systems. Also, ultraviolet light kills bugs, and there is less of it about in winter, and we tend to stay indoors more, avoiding what little there is. The risk of hypothermia is obviously greater in winter, too. These and many other seasonal effects should be considered as indirect effects of sunlight.

Aerial display

As well as melatonin, the pineal produces a range of neuro-transmitter molecules, such as 5-hydroxytryptamine, noradrena-

DEATH RATE

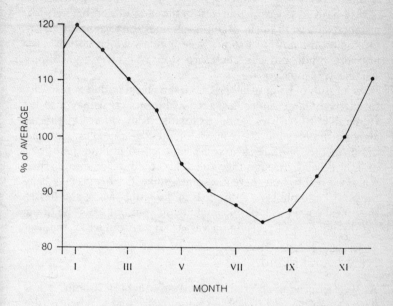

line, vasotocin and GABA.[16] It also regulates the production of certain of the endorphins – the morphine-like chemicals produced within the brain. All these chemicals have powerful effects on the way our minds and bodies function. The production rate of at least some of them is known to be influenced by dark/light cycles. So the signals from sunlight hitting the retina feed directly into some of our most crucial psychological regulatory mechnisms. There is a lot of work still to be done on finding out just how much, and in what ways, the whole brain is influenced by sunlight.

In addition to darkness and electromagnetic fields, the pineal is also open to influence from bodily hormones. In contrast to the rest of the brain, the pineal is outside the system of the cerebral ventricles, and therefore lacks a blood-brain barrier. As already explained this is a biochemical term for the filtering effect of the ventricular system of the brain, which screens out naturally occurring chemicals, as well as a number of drugs. It is very hard to get penicillin across the blood-brain barrier, for instance, and in the field of antihistamines the race has been on for some time now to produce new models which do not pass into the brain and can therefore stop you sneezing without sending you to sleep.

As a result of its unusual position, the pineal is able to respond to relatively large molecules, such as hormones. It may also be vulnerable to viruses and to toxins from micro-organisms arriving via the bloodstream.[17] Situated at the centre of the brain, in the mid-line, it may be exposed to minute quantities of light passing through the skull. This could make a little sense when we realise that there are some similarities between cells in the pineal and photoreceptor cells in the retina. More and more, the pineal comes to look like an antenna, put out from the brain for the purpose of receiving a variety of environmental signals.

New found gland

As well as producing effects directly through melatonin, it has been shown that the pineal has an influence on the whole of the endocrine system of the body. In essence melatonin suppresses production by the pituitary gland of the hormones which stimulate our other endocrine glands. This reduces the activity of the thyroid, the adrenal cortex and medulla, and the sexual organs. As well as being lower at night, our output of all these hormones it at its lowest in winter. If we weren't actually designed to hibernate in winter, we were certainly meant to take it easy!

People who live in the far north of countries such as Finland and Norway, where the winter nights are almost endless, often adapt by sleeping for very long periods in winter, but hardly at all in summer. Thus they make far fewer demands on their bodies in winter. But we have abolished night; under electric lights we can live at the same pace all year round. This sounds great, but it seems there's a price to pay.

There is also a secondary effect of the pineal, through the adrenal cortex and the thyroid, on the thymus gland, which is essential for the development and maintenance of immunity. The thymus is where all the T-cells – about which we suddenly know so much – come from. Without a functioning thymus a child would not reach adulthood, succumbing early on to infections against which he or she has no resistance. Yet this too is regulated through the pineal, and nutritionally-oriented physicians are now coming to regard sunlight as a useful component of therapy designed to stimulate a weak immune system.

Melatonin also suppresses the production of insulin by the pancreas, and therefore causes a rise in blood sugar. In contrast, calcium and vitamin D appears to stimulate the production of insulin. In full health, blood sugar is carefully regulated by the body and prevented from going either too high or too low. But low blood sugar, or hypoglycaemia, is becoming recognised as a common complaint which can trigger mood swings, migraine and even epilepsy. Here, too, sunlight plays an important part, producing regulating effects which help to keep the blood sugar stable.

In other words, there is no area of our mental and bodily functioning that the sun does not influence. Our bodies were designed to receive and use it in a wide range of ways. We were not designed to hide from it in houses, offices, factories and schools. Sunshine, reaching us through our eyes and our skin, exercises a subtle control over us from birth to death, and from head to tail.

CHAPTER 5

Vitamin D – the bone maker

If your mother ever gave you cod-liver oil capsules then you have been treated with vitamin D. In 1918 a scientist called Mellanby reported that he could cure rickets in puppies by giving them cod-liver oil. Four years later it was proved that there was a component of cod-liver oil which produced calcification and strengthening of the bones, and that this component was not vitamin A.[1] The new ingredient was labelled vitamin D. A whole generation of parents over the next few decades was very aware of the necessity to ensure adequate vitamin D intake for their growing children. Hence the unpleasant little brown capsules that so many of us were forced to swallow.

In this case, mother was right. The shift away from the land and into cities, where sunlight tends to be blocked out by buildings and pollution, has meant that our vitamin D levels are lower than they have been in the past, and particularly so in winter. The result of this, coupled with poor diet in children, was rickets.

Rickets

Rickets is returning to our inner cities, particularly in the children of immigrants, who develop it even when they eat a diet which prevented rickets when they were in their home countries. Children with rickets develop deformities of the bone that are with them for life. The long bones soften due to lack of calcium, and the child's weight causes the legs to bow outwards. The teeth are poor and fall out easily, and there is also a marked muscle weakness associated with the disease. If a girl develops rickets in childhood, she is likely to have a deformed pelvis

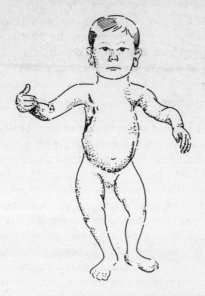

The bowed legs and arms and prominent rib joints of rickets

when she grows up; that will make childbirth difficult, and may threaten the life of both mother and child.

At the turn of the century, it was estimated that as many as ninety per cent of children in some of the crowded cities of northern Europe and the northern United States had rickets.[2] This is despite the fact that the value of sunlight and fresh air in treating rickets had been remarked on in 1822. It took an investigative committee of the British Medical Association in 1889 to state clearly that there was a relationship betwen urban industrialised environments and rickets.[3] And it was not until 1919 that it was shown that ultraviolet light could cure rickets. Over the next few years it became clear that sunlight healed or prevented rickets, and that exposing the food had this effect as well as exposing the patient; in both cases vitamin D is produced.[4] As a result, vitamin D is now added to milk and other

foods in very large quantities in the United States, with the result
that there have been problems with vitamin D overdose. In
Britain and northern Europe, however, the supplementation of
food is not required by law and is much less common, and
vitamin D levels in human beings are much lower.

Vitamin or hormone?

Although we still call it a vitamin, ih is now clear that the active
form of vitamin D is in fact a hormone, with great similarities
to the other steroid hormones – the cortico steroids produced by
the adrenal gland, which control the ability to respond to stress,
together with such basic functions as fluid balance and blood
pressure; and the androgens, oestrogens and other sex hormones
produced by the ovaries and testes which control our sexual characteristics. All of these hormones, including vitamin D, are formed in
the body from the same precursor molecule, and they all fit the
definition of a hormone: a chemical that is produced in one part of
the body and transported to another part, where it has its effect.

The necessary added ingredient to the reaction which enables
vitamin D to be formed is ultraviolet light, and for this reason
the only organ in the body that can manufacture vitamin D is
the skin. The more sunlight that reaches the skin, the more
vitamin D we produce.

The vitamin then has to go through two further chemical
conversions before it becomes active form. The first of these
happens in the liver, and the second in the kidney. Both of
these reactions are affected by hormonal and other biochemical
factors, with the result that there are a series of regulatory
mechanisms that control the level of vitamin D in the body.
This is important as it guarantees that an overdose of vitamin
D from sunlight is impossible.[5]

Calcium absorption

Although the biochemistry is complex, the major function of
vitamin D is simple. It helps the body to make efficient use of

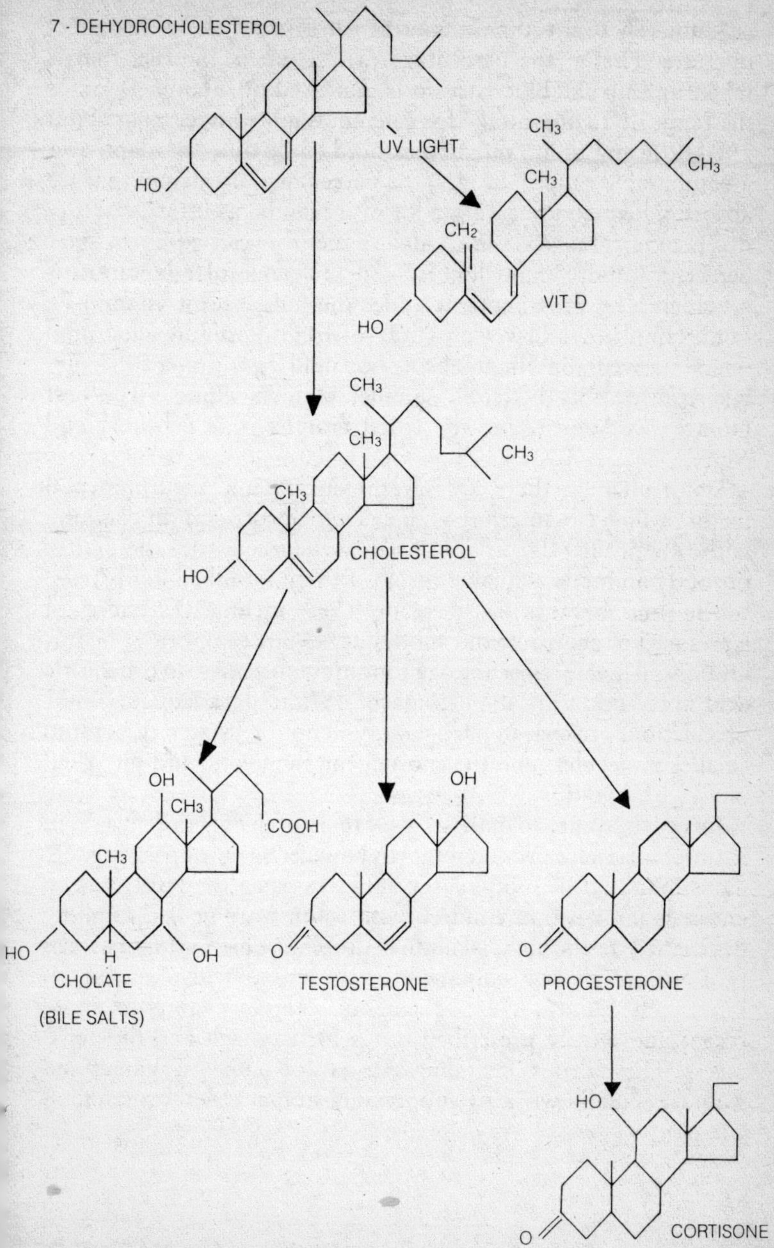

7 - DEHYDROCHOLESTEROL
HO
UV LIGHT
CH3
CH3
CH3
CH2
VIT D
HO
CH3
CH3
CH3
CH3
HO
CHOLESTEROL
OH
CH3
COOH
CH3
HO
H
OH
CHOLATE
(BILE SALTS)
OH
O
TESTOSTERONE
O
PROGESTERONE
HO
O
CORTISONE

calcium. There are three major target organs where this effect operates. Firstly, the percentage of calcium in the diet that is taken up into the bloodstream is increased by vitamin D. Since the range of dietary intake for calcium is quite large, from about 200–1200 mg daily, our bodies need to be able to adapt over a comparable range.[6] In fact, the percentage of calcium that we absorb when we are eating a lot of it may be as little as twenty five per cent, but on a low-calcium diet this can go up to sixty per cent – more than double – so the range of adaptation is considerable.[7] This happens under the influence of vitamin D. For example, a Norwegian study of healthy middle-aged prisoners showed that their absorption and retention of calcium was considerably better in summer than in winter.[8] The best month was August, and the worst months were February and March.

Unfortunately, there are several dietary and environmental factors which can interfere with calcium absorption. In common with other minerals, calcium needs to be freed from the matrix of food and made available for absorption into the bloodstream by the initial stages of digestion. These include the effects of saliva and of chewing your food, but the most important factor, and one which seems to go wrong quite often, is hydrochloric acid secretion in the stomach. Without adequate HCl production, protein, in particular, will not be broken down into smaller molecules, and the subsequent pancreatic and intestinal phases of digestion will be wasted.[9]

In old age, up to half of us can expect to be deficient in hydrochloric acid production.[10] In younger age groups, probably more than half of food-allergy sufferers have low HCl output, and it is known that children with asthma are very commonly deficient.[11] Diets high in animal protein, which contains high proportions of the sulphur-bearing amino-acids, appear to impair HCl output, as do alcohol, cannabis, and the more recent and widely prescribed drugs for stomach and duodenal ulcers. These drugs, including those trade-named Tagamet and Zantac, actually work by suppressing stomach acid production.

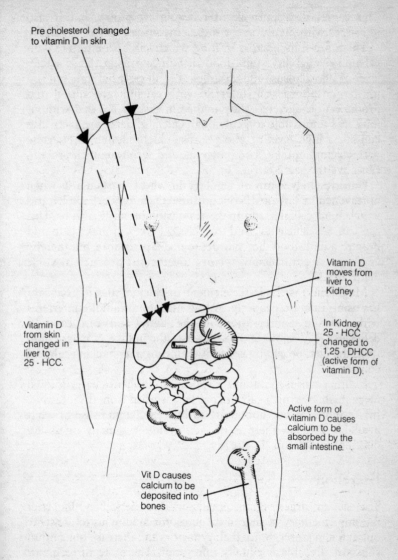

Pre cholesterol changed
to vitamin D in skin

Vitamin D
moves from
liver to
Kidney

Vitamin D
from skin
changed in
liver to
25 - HCC.

In Kidney
25 - HCC
changed to
1,25 - DHCC
(active form of
vitamin D).

Active form of
vitamin D causes
calcium to be
absorbed by the
small intestine.

Vit D causes
calcium to be
deposited into
bones

This serves their purpose of relieving symptoms, but it also interferes with digestion for these obvious reasons.

There are some factors in food which can also interfere with calcium availability. Junk-food diets in particular have a high level of phosphorus, and although it is an essential mineral, too much phosphorus can interfere with calcium absorption and produce a deficiency.[12] Despite the universal belief that without milk it is impossible to get enough calcium, dairy products also contain a high level of phosphorus – high enough to interfere with calcium uptake. Too much fat, and even too much protein, can have the same effect.

Unfortunately, bran or wholegrain wheat, particularly when unleavened or unbaked, contain some chemicals called phytates which bind calcium and make it unavailable to the body. This can cause a deficiency, and the classical error to make is to add bran to a junk-food diet in order to increase its fibre, but thereby adding two anti-calcium factors together to produce a worse deficiency.[13]

Magnesium is the sister element to calcium and is necessary for using calcium properly. A low magnesium intake interferes with calcium conservation in the body and can cause a deficiency.[14] Vitamin D also increases the uptake of magnesium from the diet, providing yet another means of enhancing calcium control.

In other words, Vitamin D appears to influence every known mechanism by which calcium can be absorbed from the intestine. It is essential if our bodies are to make maximum use of what available calcium there is in our food.[15] Yet many of us are deficient in Vitamin D already.

Excretion

The second target organ for vitamin D is the kidney. Its effect is complementary to that in the intestine, helping us to conserve our calcium stores. Since dietary factors can increase our output substantially, this is equally important. There are three major factors which do this. The first two are sugar and coffee, and both of these probably operate through the increase that they cause in the body's production of insulin. The major physiological effect of insulin is that it lowers blood sugar by pushing sugar into cells. It also pushes it into the urine, and a number of other nutrients, including amino-acids and minerals, are transported into cells or urine at the same time. A high-sugar meal or drink can increase by up to eight times the amount of calcium that we put out in our urine over the next few hours.[16] Thirdly, it appears that a diet which is high in acid residue from foods such as meat, dairy products and refined carbohydrates, as opposed to alkaline, will have a similar effect, possibly by making the urine more acid and therefore more able to dissolve calcium.

The effect of vitamin D in the kidney is simple; it causes a greater proportion of calcium (and of course of magnesium too) to be recycled back into the bloodstream rather than passed out in the urine. So not only do we absorb more of it; we also waste less.

Deposition

The third target is bone, where vitamin D increases the turnover of calcium, ensuring that more of it goes into the bones, and stays in. This means that vitamin D is essential for strong and healthy bones, not only in children, but in all age groups.

Old people, and elderly women in particular, are especially vulnerable to gradual softening of the bone due to a loss of calcium. One of the commonest problems in this age group is that people fall down and break their wrists or their hips, necessitating surgical repair of the fracture under anaesthetic.

Calcium and vitamin D are also essential for growing bones. Without them children's bones grow soft and may bend under the pressure of gravity. This is what happens in rickets. It is not just for the prevention of rickets, though, that a healthy calcium metabolism is important, but also to ensure good posture and strong bones in all children, because bones that they form in childhood will be with them all their adult life.

Teeth are also bones, of a specialised sort, and they too are dependent on calcium intake. A deficiency of sunlight, as well as calcium, can cause poor dental health and cavities in teeth.[17] When the number of dental cavities in schoolboy's mouths was surveyed in America, it was found that the more sunlight the children received, the fewer cavities they had.

Molecular messenger

The three target organ pattern described above has always led doctors to assume that the principal, if not the sole, importance of calcium is in the structure of bones. It is now known that this is far from being the case. Calcium is necessary for the functioning of every cell in the body, and there are a number of areas where its importance is starting to be appreciated.

Not only humans, of course, depend on calcium for their functioning. In this respect our metabolism is no different from that of all animals and many plants. It appears that as well as being the most abundant mineral in the body, and the chemical that gives bone its strength and its structure, calcium is a fundamental messenger between cells, of a much more primitive, early type than the sophisticated neuro-transmitters that our human brains use.[18] There is a whole category of new antihypertensive drugs called calcium channel blockers, which operate by altering the flow of calcium in and out of cells, particularly in the arteries. There has been a lot of work done to show that disorders of calcium metabolism lead also to hardening of the arteries, raised cholesterol and heart attacks.[19]

Hans Selye became famous for his description of the way that organisms adapt to stress, and without him stress would certainly not be the household word that it is. He conducted a series of experiments showing that a variety of hormones and stress factors mobilising calcium from bone into the bloodstream could lead to abnormal calcification.[20] This is a process of deposition of calcium into soft tissues so that they become hard and very like bone. It is an important part of the process of hardening of the arteries, occurring as a result of damage to the lining of the artery.

One of the major factors that can lead to abnormal calcification is an excess of vitamin D, which causes a characteristic pattern of calcified areas round joints and bones. But a deficiency of vitamin D can also lead to a rise in the level of calcium circulating in our bloodstreams. When there is more calcium than normal in the blood, it readily finds a target on which to deposit, and any local irritant or inflammation can therefore lead to abnormal calcification.

Vitamin D deficiency

Many factors influence the level of active vitamin D in our blood. The first and most important is the amount of ultraviolet hitting our skin, and therefore the amount of sunlight available and the extent to which we expose ourselves to it.

In the United States, researchers found that the average levels throughout the year for people living in Palm Beach, in sunny Florida, were twice those of people living in Seattle or Boston, a thousand miles to the north. Moreover, for both these cities, the average level in February, when vitamin D was at its lowest, was higher in men who worked outdoors than the level in August in people who worked indoors. In other words, indoor workers spend their whole lives with lower vitamin D levels than outdoor workers.[21]

When looking at American studies, one must remember that American diets are much more heavily supplemented with vitamin D than ours, and that as a consequence average vitamin D levels in America are higher all year round.

In this country, it is clear that in winter schoolchildren have less that half the vitamin D in their blood that they have in summer (January and February versus July and August), and that, even more seriously, people over sixty five may have levels throughout the winter that are less than half that of schoolchildren.[22] In these circumstances it is meaningless to talk of normals, because if everybody is deficient, then the normal levels will be deficient.

Put simply, a large proportion of this country is permanently vitamin D-deficient. The major at-risk groups are the elderly, children, pregnant and lactating mothers, and the chronically ill. Although these may not represent the majority of the population, they do amount to just about everybody who goes to see doctors. Apart from them, nobody needs a doctor! If sunlight exposure can improve the health of only a fraction of these, therefore, it can alleviate a great deal of suffering and reduce the cost to the NHS significantly.

For example, a study in Massachusetts found that ten per cent of apparently healthy elderly people were vitamin D-deficient. Of patients admitted to hospital with fractures of the hip (neck of femur), however, more than twice as many were vitamin D-deficient.[23] The study in question does not state what proportion of the patients had borderline or low normal vitamin D levels. Vitamin D clearly plays an important part in such fractures, by increasing the amount of calcium in the bones, and in these patients' cases a deficiency would appear to be at least one factor leading to their fractures.

In 1971, scientists in Boston, Massachusetts, exposed elderly men in an old soldiers' home to ultraviolet light from fluorescent full-spectrum light fixtures. The amount of added light that they received was calculated to be as much as they would get by taking a fifteen-minute walk outdoors at lunchtime in mid-summer. This was enough to improve their calcium absorption by fifty per cent compared to the control group who were under ordinary indoor lighting.[24]

The message is clear: go for a walk outside. You will raise your vitamin D levels, and at the same time the pressure of your weight on your long bones will encourage calcium to be deposited into them, making them stronger. Since this is of particular importance to old people, perhaps the most beneficial thing you can do on retirement is buy a dog!

A pain in the neck

Some of the known symptoms of vitamin D deficiency are bone and joint pain, and muscle weakness.[25] These are symptoms that are rife among the elderly and cause them to take large number of pain-killers and anti-inflammatory medications. To any general practitioner in this country, it must sometimes seem as if everybody over the age of sixty has arthritis or rheumatism of one sort or another. Of course they all expect relief from it, but the tablets that one has to offer are far from wonderful; they have to be taken constantly and they often have side effects. How much easier it would be if the sufferers could simply be offered a dose of sunlight. Nutritional practitioners nowadays often treat these problems with calcium supplements, and this is effective in many cases. Freely available solar vitamin D would achieve the same thing, with no risk of side effects and at no cost to anyone.

A study published in the *American Journal of Public Health* in 1939 showed that sunlight prevents dental caries. The researchers examined 94,000 white boys between the ages of twelve and fourteen, and they avoided pollution effects by looking only at rural areas and small towns. They found that there was a clear correlation between sunlight and caries; those boys who lived in low sunlight areas, typically in the north-eastern USA, where mean annual sunshine was less than 2,200 hours per year, had two thirds more cavities than boys living in the south-west and receiving over 3,000 hours per year.[26] Since teeth are largely made of calcium, and since calcium absorption depends on vitamin D from sunshine, this is hardly surprising.

Spacemen are fastidiously screened from any ultraviolet radiation reaching them, because of the risk of unpredictably high levels occurring. They also are known to suffer from demineralisation of the bone, with muscle weakness and general ill health as a consequence. This may be largely due to the effects of weightlessness, since pressure along the axes of the long bones is necessary to maintain their mineral content. But when a study was carried out by the Royal Navy at their Institute of Naval

Medicine in Gosport, they found that keeping young healthy males in a sunlight-free environment on the ground led to their developing serious problems within two months. By this time the vitamin D levels in their blood had gone down by half, and they were starting to lose more calcium than they took in.[27]

Unfortunately, in the true military fashion, they do not appear to have asked the subjects how they felt, so we are not told whether there were any symptoms associated with this. We do know, however, that this is precisely the sort of environment in which many chronically ill people find themselves: indoors, deprived of any ultraviolet light and with very little pressure on their long bones to stimulate mineralisation. Small wonder that when they do finally stand up their muscles and bones are weak.

When you think about it, we can add to our list of people likely to be vitamin D-deficient, anybody who has been in an English hospital for more than eight weeks. If you are having bone surgery, in other words, try not to spend too long in hospital beforehand. If you do, your bones will be weaker and take longer to heal, your heart and arteries may be at risk, and your muscles will be flabby and weak.

Before the war, both children and adults in hospital were often taken out into the sun during the day, and many hospitals were designed with verandahs and French windows to make this possible. Nowadays hospitals tend to be multi-storey, and a little like car parks too, and we have all forgotten the wisdom that was ours for free, concerning the necessity of sunlight for the elderly, children, convalescents – in fact, for every one of us.

CHAPTER 6
The big C and a little UV

Sunlight is a killer! This is the clear message from the medical profession at present. The warm, sensual feeling that you get from lying in the sun is probably immoral, and you ought to be at home taking antibiotics. Yet we persist in taking holidays in the sun, and nipping out of doors at lunchtime. Can it be that we know something the doctors don't? It definitely can, and some of the evidence to prove us right has been around for half a century. Put aside for a moment the question of skin cancer – which is dealt with in the next chapter – and think about cancers in general, which kill far more people every year.

Twenty-five years ago Dr John Ott investigated the background to a report that children at a school in Illinois had five times the national rate of leukaemia.[1] He found that the schoolhouse was a plain, modern building with very large windows in every room, and all the pupils who developed leukaemia had been in two particular classrooms. In these two rooms the teachers always kept the large curtains completely drawn across the windows to reduce glare and distraction, and to keep the children's attention on schoolwork. The indoor lighting was therefore on all the time, and this was 'warm white' fluorescent. The whole class spent its working day in light of twilight intensity, with no blue or UV light at all except at playtime – and in Illinois they have some hard winters, during which the children might not go out to play at all.

Several years later the two teachers in question left the school, and their replacements kept the classroom curtains open all the time. The lights were also replaced with cool white fluorescent ones, and of course needed to be used less. From then on there was not a single case of leukaemia in the school for as long as

Dr Ott followed it up. No other explanation has been put forward for this remarkable mini-epidemic of leukaemia; although in isolation it proves nothing, it started Dr Ott thinking about the possibility of a link between sunlight and cancer.

In fact this had been commented on half a century ago. In 1936, a report in *The Lancet* by Peller, a US Navy doctor, suggested an inverse relationship between skin cancer and all other cancers. He observed that Navy personnel had eight times the skin cancer rate of the rest of the population, but only forty per cent of the total death rate from cancer.[2] He proposed that the obvious explanation for this was the greater amount of sunlight to which men serving in the Navy were exposed. Nowadays, many naval personnel probably spend their whole working lives at computer consoles, but in 1936 they naturally led an outdoor life and were in the sun a great deal.

Peller made the startling suggestion that by using high intensities of light, either sunlight or ultraviolet from a carbon arc lamp, we should actively induce skin cancers in patients, in order to protect them from other cancers. As cancers go, those skin cancers that have been clearly shown to be related to sunlight have obvious advantages; the most important of these is that they are visible at a much earlier stage, and can therefore be dealt with. The success rate of surgery has always been good, and if you had to choose which cancer to get, skin cancer would be an excellent choice.

In fact, skin cancers cause only nine per cent of the deaths from cancer every year, and organ or internal cancers ninety one per cent. What's more, the survival rate from skin cancer is very good – about ninety five per cent of sufferers live for five years or more after diagnosis, whereas only thirty six per cent of cancer victims in general live that long. The exception, of course, is the relatively rare skin cancer called malignant melanoma, which is discussed in the next chapter.

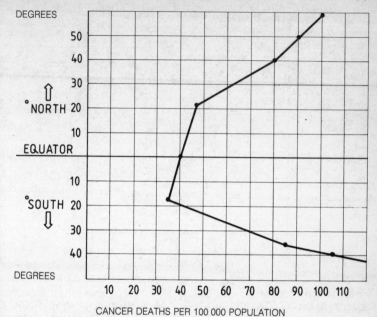

CANCER DEATHS PER 100 000 POPULATION

The global view

The really strong sunlight effect starts to show through when
you examine the relationship betweeen sunlight exposure and
cancer incidence on a global scale – the epidemiology. This has
been looked at in some detail on several occasions. The simplest
and clearest study is that performed by Hoffman for the Prudential Life Assurance Company in 1924.[3] He analysed the
frequency of cancers of all types in a total of 130 cities around
the world (looking at almost 300,000 cancer deaths) and
matched this against their latitude. The results are clearly shown
in the graph above. The further the city from the equator, the
greater the number of cancers. The ratio of highest frequency
to lowest is around 2.5 :1, which looks as though it may turn
out to be a magic figure of some sort.

This study concentrated on people living in cities, so that

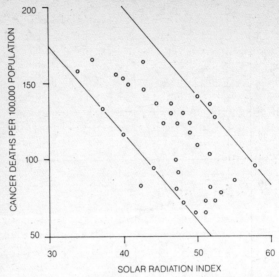

USA CANCER DEATHS DECREASE WITH RISE IN SUNLIGHT

factors such as lifestyle and levels of development should not interfere. But in 1940, when Dr Frank Apperley looked at the total mortality from cancers across the United States in both rural and urban areas, the picture he found was just the same, and very clear. He measured two factors that are likely to match closely with the average exposure of individuals to sunlight: the percentage of the population involved in agriculture (and so out of doors most of the time), and the amount of solar radiation recorded by the local Met station. He plotted these measures against the number of cancers.

This was then refined further by looking only at people over forty five (the age group in which the large majority of cancers occur), and only at the white population, who have an incidence of cancer several times higher than that of black people. Neither of these restrictions altered the results at all; the effect was the same for both methods of analysis. As you can see from the graph, the more time people are outdoors, and the more sunlight in the area where they live, the fewer cancers they develop.

Interestingly, the highest ratio comes out once again to a little over 2:1.

So what mechanisms could explain this link between light deficiency and cancer? Well, several of them. The problem with researching this kind of thing is that there is no single clearcut process involved to make it nice and easy for the scientist. Sunlight is so fundamental to our lives, and affects us in so many ways, that it may be impossible to demonstrate a single link. But we can pull several strands out of the knot, each of them a connection.

The guts of the matter

In a large North American study, higher vitamin D levels appeared to give significant protection against cancer of the colon. The analysis made was of the amount of vitamin D in the diet, not of blood levels. The researchers found that the group with the lowest vitamin D intake were about 2.5 times more likely (there's that number again) to develop bowel cancer than those with the most vitamin D in their diet.[4] We know that much of the population in this country is vitamin D-deficient for much of the year, even more so than in America. Raising people's levels of this vitamin may protect them in some way from cancer.

However, when this connection was examined in Japan, there did not appear to be the same correlation. This may be due, suggests the paper, to the fact that the Japanese, living nearer the equator, have a greater exposure to sunlight, and therefore more sunlight-derived vitamin D in their blood.[5] In these circumstances, dietary vitamin D will not be so important.

The best-known reason why vitamin D is important is that it increases our uptake of calcium from the diet. We know that calcium plays an important part in cancer of the bowel, actively calming down the rapidly dividing cells. Vitamin D will enable these cells to take up more calcium, and this may begin to explain the sunlight effect. More recently, laboratory studies have found that there are receptor sites for vitamin D on cancer cells, and that it appears capable of converting human leukaemia cells *back into normal cells* – at least in the test tube.

A breach of security

It has been estimated that we each develop cancer once a week on average. This is how often a cell in our bodies is likely to go 'rogue' and start dividing rampantly. But fortunately for us, when this happens the cell also undergoes a change in the proteins on its surface, and our immune system swiftly identifies it as 'not-self', as a threat to our health, and eliminates it. In other words, developing a cancer – a real cancer – is a sign not of something going wrong with our genes, but of something wrong with our immune systems.

This is why people with AIDS are so vulnerable to strange malignancies such as Kaposi's Sarcoma. Their immune systems are damaged by the virus, which attacks the T-cells, a type of white cell crucial to the production of antibodies against invaders. AIDS particularly kills off the T-helper cells, which are normally in balance with T-suppressor cells. T-helpers stimulate the immune system to attack, while T-suppressors discourage it from so doing. With a disproportionately low level of T-helpers the immune system is powerless against infections, cancers and other threats to our wellbeing.

Yet there are people alive in America who have had AIDS for several years but are now fit and well. They have found ways to stimulate their bodies' production of T-cells when conventional drugs were powerless to help. A variety of methods appear to have benefited them – meditation, herbs, acupuncture and megadose vitamin C among the most important.

It is now clear, from very recent studies on the skin as an immune organ, and from old studies on the effects of sunlight on the white blood cell count, that sunlight can have a dramatic effect in this area. When sunlight hits the skin, it stimulates the topmost layer of living cells, the keratinocytes. These are the cells which produce the keratin, the hard outer layer of dead skin that protects us from germs and injuries. It was always thought that they had no other function. But new evidence has proved that when they are triggered by ultraviolet light, keratinocytes produce a chemical called interleukin-1. IL-1 has a simple but potent effect: it causes white cells, and T-cells in particular, to multiply in number.

Since this is the only way that such cells can be mobilised quickly to respond to a threat, IL-1 has been the focus of considerable interest among immunologists in recent years. Despite detailed research, though, it has been clear that we are a long way from the day when we can synthesise it in a laboratory. Now there hardly seems to be any point. *Why spend millions on manufacturing something which our own bodies will make for free in response to sunlight?*

So in order to raise your white cell count, mobilise your immune system against attacks by infection or even by cancer, and absorb more protective calcium, all you need to do is sunbathe. This may help to explain why children get so many infections in winter, when we are all at risk from sunlight deficiency – and why influenza epidemics alway seem to happen then too. But it may also be an important strand in the understanding of why sunlight protects against cancer.

Free oxidising radicals

Free oxidising radicals are small negative ions with the ability to split molecules and damage cells. These atoms and small molecules with a negative charge on them are produced in chemical reactions, in the atmosphere, in food and in our bodies. Some of them are very short-lived, only existing for minute fractions of a second. However, they have a tendency to propagate rapidly, so that the production of one free oxidising radical (FOR) can, within a very short space of time, lead to a large number.

Whether single or multiple, they have a powerful ability to react with biological molecules in damaging ways. They can break open the DNA in our chromosomes, although there are mechanisms to prevent their getting near it in its safe harbour in the cell nucleus. When they do come into contact with DNA they can split it open and alter the genetic information, leading to mutations.

They also split open antibodies, the molecules used by our immune systems to attack infections and clear allergens out of the system. This can lead to effects very like allergic reactions in some people. Also, they can break open collagen molecules, the structures that make up ligaments and hold our tissues together, and give skin its elasticity. This is why pollution and smoking can age your skin.

On the other hand, free oxidising radicals are actually used by the white cells of the body to attack infecting agents. As a white cell engulfs a virus or bacterium, it pumps highly toxic FORs into the forming vacuole in order to kill the micro-organism. Thus FORs are necessary to the healthy functioning of our immune system; in other words, they are an example of something that is necessary in the right amounts, but can be toxic in overdose.

Our bodies possess a series of mechanisms for controlling FORs, mopping them up rapidly and preventing them from damaging tissues. These are known as antioxidants. The major ones are essential nutrients such as vitamins A, E, and C, the amino-acid glutathione, and certain minerals such as selenium. Some of these, such as vitamins A and E, protect by mopping up FORs themselves, so preventing them from damaging our cells. Others, such as selenium, are components of the enzymes which rapidly process and inactivate FORs. Damage produced by smoking, alcohol, radiation or even sunburn due to ultra-violet light, are all FOR effects. They are all prevented by high levels of antioxidants, in this case particularly vitamin A.

So FORs can be produced by large doses of ultraviolet light, but we can protect against this by an adequate intake of antioxidant nutrients, and by avoiding excess fat in our diet. Since we live in a light-poor environment, diet is more important in this respect than overdoses of light, with the exception of the annual jaunt to the Costa Packet. Torremolinos in summer is full of English people overdosing on sunlight, on alcohol, on greasy food, possibly on tobacco too. Along with the raffia ponies and peeling backs, they bring home a system so overloaded so rapidly that they may need the rest of the year in a dark room to recover. That we do not all develop skin cancer after our summer holidays only proves the effectiveness of the body's defences when we are in good health.

Fat and weak

Some of the molecules most vulnerable to the effects of free oxidising radicals are the oils and fats making up our cell walls, which are obtained from our diet. It is now well understood that the more oils there are in our diet the more antioxidants we need to protect them. Without these protective mechanisms, the fats may be damaged by FORs, and it is thought that their molecules may be twisted into an abnormal and highly toxic form, known as trans-fats. The greater the surplus of fats and oils over antioxidant nutrients in our bodies, the greater the probability of trans-fats being formed, and this alone may explain many cancers. Overdoses of ultraviolet light may cause this change, but only if we are short of the protective nutrients. Once again it is a matter of nutritional balance.

Despite the current powerful trend of opinion against them, it appears that saturated fats are not in themselves toxic. They do harm us, though, in two specific ways. Firstly, a high animal-fat diet may contain simply too much fat surplus, with the risk of trans-fats being formed. But polyunsaturated oils too can cause both of these damaging effects, so lashings of sunflower oil or margarine on your baked potato may be just as harmful as butter.

Secondly, saturated fats, which have no double bonds along their chain of carbon atoms, can simply replace unsaturated fats in the diet, and some unsaturated oils *are* necessary for health. The importance of unsaturation is that it means the presence of double bonds in the chemical structure of the oil. These double bonds can be opened up by enzymes and used, rather like a child's construction toy, to build new molecules. This enables the oils to be utilised by the body for cell walls and for the production of a range of other chemicals; in particular for a group of hormones called prostaglandins. Because we need a regular supply of them to process into other molecules, certain of these oils and fats are known as essential fatty acids.

Prostaglandins control a large variety of biological functions, including inflammation in response to injury or infection, the formation of blood clots in arteries and veins, and the contraction of the uterus in childbirth. Saturated fats are useless in this respect, and are therefore only able to be stored and used as calories. We need polyunsaturates for normal functioning, but the greater our intake, the more molecules we have circulating which need to be protected against FOR damage, including that from UV light.

Human studies

In 1959 Dr Ott finally had the opportunity he longed for: he was asked to participate in a study on the effects of sunlight on cancer in human patients. A physician at the Bellevue Medical Center in New York arranged for fifteen people with diagnosed cancer to organise their own sunlight therapy. Throughout the summer months, they spent as much time as possible out of doors, without any glasses or sunglasses. They also avoided artificial lights and televisions as much as possible.

When the summer ended, the physician in charge attempted to evaluate the results. She found that fourteen out of the fifteen patients had shown no further spread in their cancers, and some even appeared to have improved. The fifteenth had continued wearing spectacles, and so would have blocked ultraviolet light from entering her eyes. Although there were no controls in this experiment, and it had run for only a few months, both Dr Ott and the doctor thought that it showed sufficient effect to be worthy of further, more detailed, investigation.

The medical authorities to whom he presented these results, with a proposal for further research, thought otherwise, and no more research was done on humans. But another medical friend of Dr Ott's did become interested, and set up an experiment using a strain of mice (known as C3H mice) that are very prone to developing cancerous tumours spontaneously. He reared separate litters under pink fluorescent tubes, under 'daylight' white tubes and under sunlight. The mice under the pink tubes showed cancers first, a month before those under white tubes and three months before those in daylight.

Strangely, this study was refused for publication! Much more work will have to be done before the medical community will accept any value for light in treating cancer, and there is no sign of it being done at present. Yet the results of the small study on humans were strongly positive, and any drug company would be delighted if it would show such a positive response to their product after only a few weeks.

Take all of this evidence together and a pattern does emerge. It seems clear that we can modify our lifestyle in one simple way that will decrease our risk of developing cancer, and may even offer hope of help when we do develop it.

CHAPTER 7

The melanoma debate

1987 saw the most widespread campaign ever to try and persuade us that sunlight is dangerous and we should avoid it. Yet we still go on summer holidays in our millions, and we still come back feeling that it was worthwhile, and that we'll go again next year. Can it be that we are all so foolish that we ignore the medical evidence for the sake of two weeks of sensuality, or might our instincts be telling us the opposite of what the medical profession is telling us?

It is worth looking at the evidence with a fresh eye. For instance, everybody knows that sunlight causes skin cancer. But it is that simple? We know that cancers are much more common in hot, sunny areas such as Queensland, due to solar exposure – or do we? We all know that malignant melanoma is a skin cancer that is caused by sunburn – but is it?

The last two statements are both questionable. The first is half correct – squamous cell and basal cell carcinomas of the skin are more common in white-skinned people living in very sunny areas such as Queensland. This does not apply to cancers anywhere else in the body.[1] The last statement is, at best, misreading of the evidence. Malignant melanoma is more common in people with the sort of skin that burns easily, but we are not in a position to say that the sunburn actually causes the cancer – it may even protect against it.

We have to take all this very seriously, because in the UK one quarter of all deaths are due to cancer. There are about 200,000 new cases of cancer every year, and of these about ten per cent are skin cancers. This is turn breaks down to ninety eight per cent squamous and basal cell cancers, and two per cent melanomas.

But – and it's a very big but – the chances of surviving a skin cancer are excellent: ninety five per cent of patients are alive five years after diagnosis. This compares with thirty six per cent survival for cancers in general.[2] So, as we remarked in the previous chapter, if you have to get cancer, then skin cancer is definitely the wisest choice.

The one big exception is melanoma, of course. Although it is very rare – about 0.2 per cent of all cancers – it is the only skin cancer that normally metastasises (spreads to distant parts of the body), and the death rate is much higher. The five-year survival rate is fifty per cent, much poorer than the other skin cancers. It still doesn't rank in the top ten killers, but if it were avoidable by something as simple as staying out of the sun, this would plainly be a sensible thing for us all to do.

With the common forms of skin cancer, squamous and basal cell, the relationship with sunlight is clear. They occur usually on the exposed surfaces, such as the face, scalp and the back of the hands, usually in old age, in people who have spent many years working out in the sun. They are particularly common in people who haved lived for some time in the tropics. In other words, it is long-term steady exposure to sunlight, for several hours a day, over many years, that triggers off these cancers.

Because it is so much less common, it has been much harder to gather sound evidence on melanoma and its relationship to sunlight. But until recently, a single fact was always quoted as proof that it was triggered by sun. This was the particularly high incidence of melanoma in Queensland, in Northern Australia. This is one of the hottest and sunniest places on earth, and it seemed that the link was obvious and inescapable.

Yet when studies were done in Queensland itself, it was found that within the state boundaries, the sunnier the area the fewer melanoma cases occurred. The disease was more common in the coastal areas, which had less sunlight in summer, when the amount of UV was higher. This clearly bemused the doctors doing the research, as they had no other explanation for melanoma than damage from UV.[3]

The next episode in the story also occurred in Australia, with a survey in New South Wales which showed that there was a greater risk of melanoma in women who had been exposed to fluorescent light at work than in those who have not. The longer these women had been working under fluorescent lights, the greater their risk of developing the cancer. Sunlight appeared to play no significant part in causing the problem.[4]

Critics of this study said that this might be a false result due to the fact that people of a higher social class were more prone to melanoma, and also – but incidentally – were more likely to work in offices with fluorescent lighting. But a study in the New York area confirmed the finding in a group who were all predominantly middle class. With no difference between the social class of the melanoma sufferers and the non-sufferers, fluorescent lights still appeared to increase the risk.[5]

That was in 1982. In 1984 a large study of 507 melanoma cases and 507 matched controls (matched for age, sex and place of residence) was performed in Western Australia. This one found that, if anything, exposure to sunlight protected against melanoma. People who regularly spent ten hours a week or more in the sun had a lower chance of developing the disease, and the longer time they spent in the sun each week the lower their risk. There *was* an increase of melanoma in people who went boating or fishing twice a week, but this was more than the increase in those who sunbathed – hardly strong evidence of a sunlight link. In fact, the worse a person's history of sunburn in the past, the less the chance of their developing at least one type of the cancer, known as nodular melanoma.[6]

The final piece of research, which looks as though it may have made sense of the whole conundrum, was conducted in Canada in 1985. This showed that the real risk came not from sunburn, but from having the type of skin that burnt easily. Whether or not a person actually got sunburned was not important in comparison to their tendency to burn easily and tan poorly. Those with the most sensitive skin had twice the risk of melanoma of those who never burned.[7]

Despite all this, the Royal College of Physicians Report published in April 1987 still said that sunlight was the culprit in melanoma.[8] The conclusion was largely based on the research of one doctor in Glasgow who found a high proportion of people with a history of bad sunburn in her study. She took no account, however, of the point made by the Canadian study, that people who burn badly are likely to have sensitive skin – and of course in Scotland a very high proportion of the populace has Type One, or Celtic, skin. They may never tan, only develop freckles, and the lack of melanin in their skin makes them very susceptible to sunburn.

There are several small points that round out this argument. Firstly, studies in the laboratory show that vitamin D suppresses malignant melanoma – and also leukaemia – in test tube experiments.[9] Understandably, no one is attempting to reproduce this in humans, but it does offer a possible explanation for the apparent protective effect of regular sunlight against melanoma.

Secondly, the ultraviolet wavelengths that produce vitamin D in the skin are entirely absent from normal fluorescent lighting – and the total UV exposure from working under fluorescent lights for a year has been calculated to be equivalent to about forty minutes of autumn sun.[10] So how can UV be the culprit?

Thirdly, the incidence of malignant melanoma is going up most rapidly in some far from tropical areas such as Scandinavia and Scotland. It has been estimated to be doubling approximately every ten to twenty years.[11] Nobody has yet shown how this increase could be due to exposure to sunlight. But it could very well be due to increasing exposure to indoor lighting.

Finally, despite the recommendations in the RCP report, there is evidence that sunscreens make no difference to the incidence of melanoma. Indeed, there has been for some time proof that they may even contribute to causing skin cancer, as well as certainly helping to trigger off photosensitivity – skin rashes in response to sunlight.[12]

When Apperley, who showed that cancers in general decreased with sunlight exposure, looked at the incidence of skin cancer throughout the continental USA, he found that the relationship with sunlight depended on the average temperature. Over a critical level of 42°C, increases in exposure to sunlight clearly caused an increase in the rate of development of skin cancers – of all types. Below that temperature, however, the rate decreased with increasing exposure to sun.[13]

It would appear, then, that in hot, tropical countries there is a risk of sunlight causing skin cancer, particularly in white skins, of course. In temperate climates such as northern Europe, on the other hand, sunlight is likely to protect. This would also tie in with the finding that, in contrast to Panner's figures mentioned in the last chapter, English researchers have found that rates of skin cancer and total cancers vary together.[14] In temperate climates such as ours, sunlight may protect us from both skin cancers and cancers in general, while in hot climates it may encourage skin cancers (basal cell and squamous cell), but still protect against other cancers.

The overall picture, then, seems to be that sunlight in large doses for long periods may cause skin cancer, particularly in the tropical heat, but sunlight at any dose level protects from cancers in general. The more sunlight you receive, the better protected you are. We know that sunburning with its production of free oxidising radicals is the factor that encourages the development of skin cancer. There is no reason to think that this is the protective factor against other cancers, so the way to take your sunlight as a cancer protection is in frequent small doses, insuf- fient to burn you. The secretary who slips out of the office at lunchtime and sunbathes in the park for forty minutes has the right idea. As well as gorgeous brown legs, she is giving herself protection against cancer.

Atmospheric filter

The wavelengths that are responsible for sunburn are those with the highest energy content – ultraviolet. Because their wave- length is shorter, there are more waves per metre of length, or per second, hitting the skin, and therefore more energy is transferred. Compared to ultraviolet, infra-red has a very low energy content. The whole of our biology is based round the

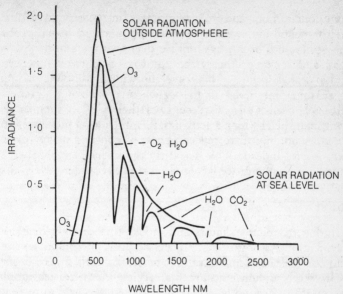

THE SOLAR RADIATION AT SEA LEVEL IS THE RESULT
OF ABSORPTION BY MOLECULES IN THE ATMOSPHERE

fact that there is a very sharp cut-off point for ultraviolet transmission through the atmosphere.

There are two gateposts framing the narrow inlet for solar radiation. On the low frequency, long wavelength side, much of the solar spectrum is absorbed by carbon dioxide and water, while on the short wavelength side the most important absorber is ozone. It is the fact that ozone absorbs best at a wavelength of 260 nanometres, and the absorption then tails off completely above 300, that gives us the cut-off point for solar radiation at around 300 nanometres.

There has been concern among scientists in recent years about the danger that certain environmental pollutants, particularly the propellants in aerosol cans, may destroy the ozone layer in the atmosphere and lead to an increase in the amount of ultraviolet reaching the earth. However, the ozone level varies greatly from hour to hour and from day to day, in response to normal environmental and weather factors. The level of ozone in the atmosphere has been measured for over fifty years in the Swiss Alps, and in some other places, and no clear trend has been demonstrated so far.[15] This is true notwithstanding the finding of an apparent 'hole' in the ozone layer above Antarctica. Although such a discovery suggests that our environment is being disturbed by man's activities, it is still a local phenomenon and does not appear to reflect a general reduction in the ozone layer – yet. Indeed, some scientists think that it may always have been there and we have only just noticed it.

Smog

Pollution from car exhausts and industry produces a range of chemicals in the atmosphere, including both the components of acid rain (sulphates and nitrates in particular), and indeed ozone itself. In this circumstance, with a very high local concentration at just above ground level, ozone is more important as a toxic pollutant than as a sunscreen. In fact, the level of ozone in smog appears to be increased by ionisation triggered by ultraviolet light. Monitoring of the intensity of sunlight in Washington DC and California has shown a *reduction* in the sunlight reaching the earth of more than ten per cent over the last fifty years, with a twenty six per cent reduction in the ultraviolet fraction.[16] The only evident cause of this is environmental pollution.

Therefore, if you live under a smog, as many people in cities around the world now do, you receive less ultraviolet light because it is absorbed by the smog. You also breathe less fresh air and more pollution. Once again, modern life has increased the toxic component of our intake while reducing the nutritional or beneficial component. In this case, it appears that ultraviolet light helps to make the problem worse by interacting with the chemical components of smog. But the real culprit is not the ultraviolet light, it is the products of fossil fuel combustion that go to make up pollution.

Photoreactivation

It is ultraviolet light of around 295 nanometres wavelength (UVB) which has the potential to cause damage to DNA and other molecules. These are the shortest wavelengths – and therefore have the highest energy – of any light reaching the earth. Thus they have the greatest potential for transferring energy to our bodies – for producing either benefit or damage.

Damaged DNA may lead to a cellular mutation – an abnormal cell which can be the start of cancer, or in the next generation of a genetic change or a congenital abnormality. Although several people have suggested that this is necessary for evolution, that an element of randomness is needed to keep things changing, it is certain that the process does lead to cancers and deformities. Under normal circumstances, all such genetic mutations are filtered out of the body by the immune system.

When cancer develops this is detected at an early stage by the immune surveillance and the cells are killed and removed. Clinical cancer is therefore more a sign of an immune problem than of something unusual in the way of genetic events. Transplant patients who have received immunosuppressant drugs so that they will not reject the transplanted heart or kidney have an *eighty times greater* than normal chance of developing cancer. Victims of the AIDS virus also have a tendency to develop unusual forms of cancer such as Kaposi's Sarcoma. Both groups have in common a low level of immunity to infections and to cancers.

But it has always been known that some organisms have the ability to repair DNA damage in a manner that is dependent on ultraviolet light. Many micro-organisms have been shown to contain a protein molecule – an enzyme – which absorbs near-ultraviolet light (UVA), and is thereby activated to repair broken strands of DNA. [17]

The chemicals that are measured as an indicator of DNA damage are known as pyrimidine dimers. These are small component molecules of DNA which have been broken free of the chromosome and then joined together in pairs to form dimers (which consist of two identical molecules). Evidence of repair of DNA damage is obtained if these dimers are split into two monomers again. The process by which this occurs in response to UV light is called photoreactivation. It has always been known that it occurs in small organisms, but until recently it was thought that higher animals did not perform this function. In the past decade there has been increasing evidence that it occurs in a range of mammals, and the hunt was therefore on for evidence of its occurence in humans.[18]

In 1986 Betsy Sutherland, a researcher at Brookhaven National Laboratory in New York, finally demonstrated that photoreactivation occurred in human skin. She described its parameters quite clearly: it is light-dependent, being stimulated best by light of wavelength 350 to 400 nanometres, which is in the near ultraviolet range. When such light hits the skin, the process happens very rapidly, clearing most of the dimers out of the tissue within minutes.[19]

There is also some non-enzymatic repair that is still dependent on light, but occurs by chemical reactions that do not depend on human enzymes. Although this can be measured in skin also, it occurs at a much slower rate, taking about an hour to remove half of the dimers. Clearly it is less important than photoreactivation.

The remarkable fact is that although ultraviolet stimulates the synthesis of DNA, and therefore cell activity and multiplication, it suppresses DNA synthesis during the first hour after exposure.[20] During this hour, the photoreactive enzymes are able to repair most of the damaged DNA in readiness for the burst of cellular activity that then occurs. Therefore, as well as having a potential for damaging human tissues, ultraviolet light is also essential for the repair of such damage. We are so well adapted to our solar environment that there is a built-in protective mechanism, triggered by sunlight, to protect us against the possible harmful effects of this same sunlight.

The message seems clear. Although some doctors and scientists are still determined to prove that sunlight is damaging and should be avoided, the evidence is mounting in its favour. We are designed to feed on sunlight, and we suffer if starved of it. But changes in our lifestyle over the past few decades have only advanced a process started by the industrial revolution, driving us indoors and away from the sun. Attemping to rectify this by brief binges of sunlight for a fortnight in the summer may well have harmful effects that offset their benefits. *We should aim to nourish ourselves with sunlight regularly, every week of the year.*

CHAPTER 8
Invisible radiations

One of the more ironic aspects of science is its ability to deceive itself into believing that scientific progress is reasonable, logical and inexorable. Scientists are taught that the 'scientific method' – the process laid down for the development of scientific knowledge – has the power and status of a force of nature. Careful observation of the available facts is followed by the formulation of a hypothesis. An experiment is set up to prove or disprove this hypothesis, and the results lead to the development of a better hypothesis, and a new experiment, and so on.

Unfortunately, this does not always work. Many ideas are stillborn because scientists, being only human, find it difficult to consider something that does not meet their preconceptions. Others die young, because a new and more exciting discovery is made which pushes them out of the spotlight of scientific interest. Such a fate, it seems, befell the study of the phenomenon of invisible radiation by organisms, which we shall now call bioradiation. It remains unheard of by most scientists, and the advances in technology since it was first described have hardly been applied to thoroughly examining and proving or disproving it. Yet its implications are so great that it could change all our lives radically.

The living wave

For some years now we have known that the Russians are many years ahead of the West in their investigation of telepathy, psychokinesis and paranormal phenomena of every sort, together with the Eastern disciplines of acupuncture, traditional Chinese medicines and herbs. So it has been with bioradiation.

Although in the thirties there were a number of studies in Europe and America, it is in Russia that all the donkey-work has gone on. Dozens of papers have been produced, and the baton of research has passed down to sucessive generations of the same family which made the breakthrough over sixty years ago. Indeed, the Russians still publish on bioradiation; the most recent study I can find was published in 1982, by a descendant of Alexander Gurwitsch.[1]

In 1923 Gurwitsch found that he could stimulate the growth of cells, and their division, by exposing them to radiations from an already growing organism.[2] In his first experiments, he used onion roots. These were arranged in glass tubes enveloping most of their length, so that only the parts needed in the experiment were exposed. On the side of the detector root nearest to the transmitter root, more cells divided, and there was an increase in size and chemical activity.

His first assumption, or hypothesis, was that this was due to a chemical substance released from the transmitter root. So he inserted a quartz sheet between the two roots to block any such mediators, and found that the effect was not abolished. When a sheet of glass was interposed instead, however, there was no response by the detector root. Since the effect could pass through quartz, it had to be an electromagnetic wave; but if it could not pass through glass, then it was almost certainly in the ultraviolet part of the spectrum.

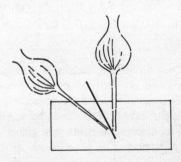

Life monitor

Over the next decade this experiment was repeated in a variety
of different organisms, ranging from staphylococcus bacteria,
through yeasts and plants, to human blood, excised human
cancers and bone marrow.[3] All of them showed biological radiation. However, the tissues of animals or humans that were near
to death did not show any radiation. Nor, it seemed, did any
human tissues with the exception of brain, blood and muscle.
It was several years before later, more carefully designed, experiments showed that all tissues radiate, but some of them at a
much lower intensity than others.[4]

The degree of radiation appeared to depend on what was
going on in the organism or tissue. Cells which were in the
process of growing and dividing radiated most, and cells in a
state of exhaustion radiated least. In fact, the radiation detected
from human blood was highest when the individual's energy
level was high, and at its lowest after a day's hard work. Blood
from anybody with a serious illness did not radiate well, and
the most dramatic difference was found with cancer patients.

The lack of any radiation from the blood of people with
cancer was so striking that the researchers came to regard this
as a reliable test for cancer, and many cases of previously undiag-
nosed cancer are reported to have been detected by this method.[5]
When they took samples from the malignant growth itself, on
the other hand, they found that it radiated very strongly. They
reported that it seemed as though the cancer had all the vitality
and had somehow taken it away from the rest of the body.

Atomic power

The background to mitogenetic radiation is simple biochemistry
and physics. An atom is made up of a nucleus in the centre,
around which electrons orbit in fixed patterns – at least this is
one of the conflicting explanations used by science. When electrons are moved from orbit to orbit they either emit or absorb
electromagnetic radiation. The wavelength of this radiation is

precisely linked to the orbit of the electron; it has to contain exactly the right amount of energy to shift the electron from orbit A to orbit B – no more and no less. For many of the common biochemical reactions in the human or any other living body, the wavelengths fall within the ultraviolet.

When this radiation is passed from one living cell to another, it appears to be able to stimulate the very same set of chemical reactions in the receiving cell. In fact, the pattern of wavelengths emitted by any one cell can be regarded as a distinctive bioradiation 'fingerprint'.[6] It would certainly enable us to determine the precise origin of the cell, and probably also its state of health and functioning. It will also, naturally, produce the best response in cells of the same type as itself, and may even be damaging to cells of different species.

It is this property that may enable bioradiation to control the growth and development of a plant root, for instance, keeping it distinct and successful despite all the different cells from different organisms that surround it. It could, perhaps, enable bioradiation to determine the whole course of development of the embryo of a frog, a camel or a human from unicellular organism into finished animal.

The next key finding was that bioradiation could be triggered off by exposing cells to a source of ultraviolet light. When a carbon-arc lamp, the 'black light' familiar from detective stories, which was the only source of UV available in laboratories at that time, was directed at a preparation of cells, they not only

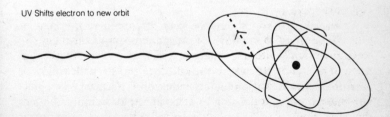

UV Shifts electron to new orbit

produced their own bioradiation in response, but an increase in metabolic activity followed as well. The implication is clear: UV from natural, sunlight sources must be equally able to stimulate our metabolisms.

Radiating health

The progress of such work in the early years was slow. In order to measure the amount of energy emitted at different wavelengths from a single chemical process, it was necessary to do a series of single experiments, each allowing through only a small waveband. The energy transmitted through a narrow-band light filter was measured by assessing how much growth it stimulated in a suspension of organisms. Alternatively, the increase in a chemical reaction could be measured. Nowadays it is possible to measure the energy directly, using a photo-electric cell.[7]

Despite these constraints, two remarkable properties of bio-radiation were discovered. The first is that the secondary radiation (the energy put out by an organism or solution in response to an input of ultraviolet energy) became stronger the more dilute the solution. Thus a 0.02 per cent solution of nucleic acid produced its peak effect in one fifth of the time taken by a 1 per cent solution. Similar results were found with suspensions of bacteria.[8]

This, of course, is very reminiscent of the response pattern of homoeopathic remedies. It is interesting to speculate that there might be a connection between bioradiation and homoeopathy. It might bring us a step nearer to understanding this mysterious and paradoxical therapy.

Acupuncturists too should be very interested in the field of bioradiation, as the whole of acupuncture is based on the concept of invisible 'chi' energy, which is essentially the life force. They say that 'where the chi goes the strength follows', meaning perhaps that biological radiation is necessary to stimu-late the growth and division of cells, and their continued effec-tive functioning. Certainly, it was realised by the early researchers that one of the most effective ways of getting a cell to radiate was to traumatise it mechanically; and the principal treatment method in acupuncture is the insertion of tiny needles through the skin, which will definitely traumatise the cells that are hit. Perhaps the whole therapeutic effect of acupuncture is mediated through bioradiation.

A further remarkable property of bioradiation is that of amplification. When six quartz test tubes containing bacteria were set side by side, and the first one was irradiated with UV, there was a secondary radiation emitted from the other end of the row, which was twenty seven times greater than the input UV.[9] This means that any living organism may be able to act as an amplifier that intensifies the signal as it is transmitted through its cells. Bioradiation is not something that can be transmitted over long distances from one human or animal to another, for good or damaging effect. When radiating through a gas or liquid devoid of life, bioradiation will soon be dispersed and wasted without effect. But within our bodies, even in response to an appropriate stimulus from outside, it may turn out to be one of the most powerful life forces there are.

We can take in the relevant energy in the most simple and primal method, known to all organisms. We can sunbathe. This allows the blood as it passes through the capillaries in the surface of the skin to be gently bathed in ultraviolet and all other wavebands of light. The energy thus obtained can be transported in the red blood cells, and emitted over the next few days.[10]

There are far too many beneficial effects from sunlight exposure for them to be entirely explained by the pineal effects and vitamin D synthesis. Bioradiation could provide an explanation for much of this, and enable us to start to make sense, at last, of man's psychological and physical need for sunlight.

CHAPTER 9
Intravenous sunlight

In 1928 a sensational new technique was introduced, which looked like revolutionising medical practice. This simple treatment appeared to be able to cure many severe and even terminal bacterial infections rapidly. It succeeded in killing viruses that were unresponsive to any other therapy, and cleared toxins from the blood within days that might otherwise have been fatal. What was more, it appeared to increase the oxygen-carrying capacity of the blood by 50 per cent, and to cure a number of conditions, from asthma through paralytic ileus (a failure of the bowel activity) to thrombophlebitis, that were otherwise untreatable. Yet ten years later, penicillin was discovered, and a few years later this therapy had sunk without trace.

The technique was straightforward: ultraviolet irradiation of the blood. A needle was inserted into a vein to remove blood, which was passed through a treatment machine and a pump, then back into the same vein, in a manner almost identical to modern kidney dialysis machines. The treatment component was very different, however. In a chamber within the irradiation machine, blood was exposed for a controlled time and intensity to ultraviolet light from a mercury-quartz bulb.[1]

Light transfusion

Much of the work on developing this treatment was done at the Hahnemann Medical College in Philadelphia. This medical school was established to train doctors in conventional medicine, but with homeopathic skills. Throughout the 1930s and 40s, thousands of patients were treated with light tranfusion. Even where contemporary chemotherapy had proved quite ineffective, the Knott technique, as it came to be known, after Dr E. K. Knott, who refined the therapy, produced dramatic results. The lives of many patients with bacterial infections were saved, including cases with generalised septicaemia who were near to death.[2] These results are very similar to those achieved with the most modern and sometimes intravenous antibiotic therapy nowadays – and they carried none of the ill effects that we now know antibiotics to have.

The one disease that did not respond to treatment with light transfusion was a severe infection involving the heart called bacterial endocarditis. Even now, this is regarded as a grave illness with a serious risk of mortality, and a high proportion of damage to the heart in those patients who survive. Unless treated rapidly and vigorously, patients invariably die.

Even more exciting, particularly to us in the 1980s, is the effect that was achieved with viral infections. Doctors treating a range of infections from viral pneumonia, through mumps to acute poliomyelitis, found that the illness cleared within days, and the abnormal temperature, blood cell counts and physical signs were corrected.[3] This achievement has yet to be matched by modern medicine. Antibiotics are ineffective against viruses, and although there are several antiviral drugs on the market now, none of them has an effect which could be termed dramatic – except by advertising copywriters.

All of this becomes especially important in the light of the contemporary AIDS crisis. Because scientific medicine has no effective treatment for AIDS, many people who find that they have the infection are paralysed by fear, which can destroy their will to fight the disease and may even damage their immune system directly. This can only accelerate their deterioration and death. If ultraviolet light in any shape or form offers hope of effective treatment for viruses, including AIDS, then we should examine it urgently.

In 1986 I visited the St Petersburg, Florida, clinic of Dr William Philpott, who is one of the most respected physicians practising nutritional medicine in the world today. He has, in collaboration with some German workers, developed a technique of ozone therapy which has striking similarities to the Knott technique. About 250 ccs of blood is removed from a vein and mixed with ozone, produced by a commercial ozone generator such as may be found in laboratories and in swimming pool treatment plants. The blood is then returned to the body through an ordinary intravenous drip.

It has been known for years that ozone can replace chlorine in swimming pools. Ozone has an even better profile of cleansing and germ-killing effects; it has no unpleasant odour and does not irritate the eyes – not to mention that some people develop allergies to chlorine. Dr Philpott says that by injecting ozone intravenously we are applying a powerful oxidising agent, and micro-organisms are at least ten times more vulnerable to oxidation than humans. So as well as boosting oxygen levels in the blood, ozone therapy should kill off infections directly.

These effects are clearly similar to those of the Knott technique. There may well be similarities between the two mechanisms, such as that part of the impact of the Knott technique is through oxidative effects of ultraviolet light. However, we have the evidence of the work of Gurwitsch and others on ultraviolet transmission by cells or 'bioradiation'.[4] From this it is clear that intake of ultraviolet light can have powerful effects on metabolism and on health. It *can* stimulate oxidation – and also reduction, glycolysis, proteolysis and a range of other enzymatic processes. It can cause cells to divide and multiply, accelerating wound healing, stimulating the release of new blood cells from the bone marrow and encouraging the production of cells and of antibodies by the immune system. Ultraviolet irradiation of the blood, either by the Knott technique or by simple exposure of the skin to sunlight, nourishes and heals our bodies – like the food that it is.

Germicidal light

In 1877 two scientists called Downes and Blount reported in the *Proceedings of the Royal Society* that sunlight had the effect of killing bacteria.[5] Their chance observation arose when solutions of sugar water left on the windowsill became cloudy in the shade, but remained clear in the sunlight. When the two solutions were examined under a microscope there were bacteria growing in the cloudy one, which had been in the shade, but none in the sunlight-exposed tube.

Over the next thirty years it was established that the ultraviolet component of the solar spectrum had this effect, and that it was effective in killing off a number of the most important micro-organisms then known to science. These included anthrax, cholera, dysentery, the plague and tuberculosis. In 1903 the Nobel prize was awarded to Niels Finsen for his demonstration that sunlight therapy could treat tuberculosis of the skin. Within a few years sunlight was also being used for tuberculosis anywhere in the body, and a number of sanatoria were set up, in the countryside of England and other nations, but especially in the Swiss Alps, to treat tubercular patients by this method. By all accounts, their results were good.

In the air

A sufficient dose of ultraviolet will kill any living cell.[6] That is why spacemen have to be protected from it. However, only a fraction of this UV reaches the earth's surface. Seasonal and weather factors come into play too; there is between two and two and a half times as much sunlight in summer as in winter. Also, the shorter the wavelength, the more the light is scattered by the atmosphere, and UV has the shortest wavelength of any light reaching the earth. As a result the summer/winter ratio climbs with UV of wavelengths below 350 nanometres to a factor of four, and below 300 nanometres there may be no radiation around in winter at all.[7]

Nevertheless, there should be enough UV in sunlight all year round, on average, to kill the large majority of bacteria and moulds within an hour. Just as lichen only grows on the northern sides of trees, so micro-organisms have to find dark and preferably damp places in which to thrive. Moulds in houses require a certain percentage of humidity in order to survive at

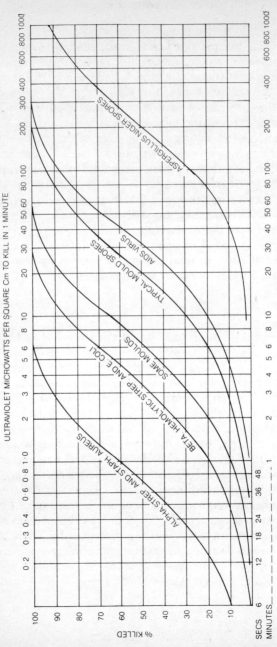

all, and of course sunlight dries them out. Wet bacteria and moulds are about four times more resistant to ultraviolet killing than dry ones.

As the diagram shows, all bacteria and moulds are susceptible to killing by UV. Viruses have a wider range of susceptibility, some of them being inactivated by the same amount of UV that kills bacteria, but others being up to two hundred times more resistant. Nevertheless, if you can give them enough, it will kill them.

The AIDS virus has approximately the same sensitivity as most moulds. Nearly all toxins, such as those excreted from staphylococcus, diphtheria, and tetanus organisms, are also inactivated by UV – as are, remarkably enough, all snake venoms.[8] This does not mean that we can use UV to inactivate them once they are inside the body; we can't guarantee light reaching that far. But it does mean that in areas that are subject to dampness or mould, or where infection is a serious problem, UV can be used to kill the organisms.

Building with light

In Sweden, every building must have adequate nuclear fall-out shelters for all the people in it. Consequently all new homes and offices – even churches – have large cellars with several feet of concrete protection and heavy lead-lined doors. Naturally these rooms are used normally for a variety of purposes – as storage, or meeting rooms, for example. But in the long cold Scandinavian winters, the problems with lighting and ventilation can lead to a build-up of mould in underground rooms. Swabbing down with bleach or other chemicals can often kill the mould, but without inactivating the mycotoxins that they produce, which may linger and continue to cause damage to health. For this reason, health campaigners in Sweden have become interested in using full-spectrum lighting in such rooms, in order to kill the moulds and destroy their toxins simultaneously, as well as providing a healthy form of illumination.

Since most organisms get into our body from the air, and

in dust on the skin, environmental ultraviolet light is clearly important in keeping down the rate of human infection in general. Out of doors this will happen naturally, but within buildings it may be necessary to use an artificial source of UV. There have been a number of studies that have shown that this works. One in school classrooms in Uppsala, Sweden, found that the bacterial count in the air went down 50 per cent when UV lights were installed;[9] the same effect was found in a US Navy barracks.[10] Both of these studies also found that the rate of infection among the children or the recruits went down by between about twenty five per cent year-round, and by thirty five per cent in winter, at the peak time for such infections. On the other hand, a study on students at the University of Illinois found as much as a fifty per cent reduction in colds when the subjects themselves, rather than the air they lived in, was exposed to UV light.[11]

Sad to say, Russia is the only country that appears to be making wise use of this effect now; ultraviolet light is used in schools and factories to improve fitness and reduce infections throughout the winter.[12] The amount of unnecessary suffering that is caused by our failure to perceive and use these health effects of ultraviolet light is preposterous.

Surgical intervention

In 1935 it was shown that using ultraviolet lights in a surgical operating theatre could kill all bacteria within ten minutes, even though it would take one and a half hours for the most sensitive skin to go red.[13] Over the next five years, surgeons at the Duke Medical Center in North Carolina published several papers on the use of UV in decontaminating the air in the operating theatre. They found that the number of airborne bacteria was cut by over fifty per cent.[14]

Subsequent studies found that it was also possible to reduce the rate of postoperative infection by about fifty per cent – although only in certain groups of operations. This probably makes sense; it would be absurd to suggest that other factors, such as the general health of the patient, did not play a part. To this day there are some surgical teams in America and Canada who still use UV light, especially in orthopaedic and neurological procedures, where an infection can have devastating results. They remain persuaded that it helps to reduce the problem.[15] And nobody has found any evidence that it harms the health of patients or staff in any way – which is more than can be said for antibiotics.

The overuse of antibiotics appears to have bred a new generation of superbugs which are resistant to nearly all available antibiotics. This has led to a lucrative race between drug companies to produce newer and more lethal antibiotics. Unfortunately, there is no sign of a cure to the problem yet. If hospitals installed low-intensity ultraviolet lights and left them on for most of the day, they might well achieve a major reduction in this problem. The fact that they would improve the health of their patients in several other ways at the same time would simply be a bonus.

On the skin

The second level of defence is on the surface of the skin itself, and is due to the same free oxidising radicals as in ozone therapy, but in a different form. In this case it is the lipids or oils in the skin which provide the oxidising effect. In 1936 an elegantly simple experiment showed that when skin was exposed to ultraviolet light for eight hours, the 'active oxygen content' went up by 10-15 fold.[16] It was then demonstrated that a large part, at least, of this oxygen was in the skin lipids or fats. These lipids were sufficiently 'active' to fog a photographic plate, and they killed haemolytic streptococcus, a relatively nasty microorganism, in just a few hours. When a solution of cysteine, which is a well-known antioxidant nutrient, was added to the experiment, then the killing effect was slowed down but by no means abolished.[17] We know from this that it was an effect due to free oxidising radicals. The same effect was achieved with the skin lipids, of course, by exposing them to ozone.

It seems that even without ultraviolet light, skin lipids will take up some oxygen from the air and use it to kill bacteria. However, this effect is much more intense under UV. Since ultraviolet light or sunlight will have a direct effect itself by killing off the organisms on and near the skin, there is clearly a double impact in this layer of defence. But both components are lost to those who stay indoors, for example in hospitals, or who cover their wounds with bandages and dressings. It would appear to make more sense for the nurses to wheel patients outside into the fresh air and remove their dressings to expose them to whatever sunlight there may be.

Now that we have conquered the majority of bacteria (outside hospitals, that is) the two infective agents that are causing the most problems are viruses, from AIDS to influenza, and fungi. Chronic fungal skin infections such as athlete's foot and ringworm are a continuing problem, but the real growth area is an organism called candida. We have known for forty years that direct ultraviolet light kills viruses and fungi. In this country we have never fully applied this discovery.

Usually thought of simply as the organism that causes a vaginal infection called thrush, candida came to prominence when it was found that it could also cause generalised infections in patients whose immune systems had been suppressed in order to allow a transplant to take. Although severe for the sufferers, this problem is small in volume. But it is now becoming clear, thanks to the work of Drs Orion Truss and William Crook in the United States, that candida is a much bigger problem.[17] Due to the increased use of antibiotics, not only to control infections but often in agriculture to prevent infections of stock animals, it is likely that we all now carry a level of antibiotic in our blood.

As well as killing off pathogenic (damaging) organisms, antibiotics also kill off the normal organisms that live in our bowel and are necessary for the process of digestion and absorption of food. It is at such moments that the candida and other fungal infections, which are less inhibited by antibiotics, can breed in the gut. When it gets a foothold in this way, candida can become a chronic problem and have a damaging effect on the immune system. It is certainly one of the factors, and maybe one of the important ones, that contribute to people who carry the AIDS virus developing the full AIDS syndrome.

One of the notable characteristics of candida infections is that they are often worse in humid conditions (fungi need humidity in order to survive) and in winter, when less light is available. Sunlight therapy can have a dramatic curative effect on athlete's foot and other skin fungi.[18] It also appears to be beneficial in many cases of candida infection, and in post-viral syndrome. Clearly it can be a valuable ally in the fight against fungus.

We know that sunlight helps to protect us from infective organisms at three levels: in the air, on our skin and within our bodies. *We are not dealing here with a chance effect of solar radiation but with a major part of the fabric of our world, and one on which we depend in many different ways. If we ignore it or shun it, we do so at our peril.*

CHAPTER 10

Acquired immune efficiency

With the discovery – or is it the invention? – of photo-immunology, we now have to realise that the skin is one of the most important organs of the body. Apart from the fact that we live through our skin – we feel with it, we kiss with it, we give off visual and odour signals with it – the skin is an essential part of the immune system. It appears that there are several different types of cells in the skin which trigger immune responses. The existence of these cells has only been known about for half a dozen years, so we certainly do not have a detailed picture of how they interact. We know enough to appreciate that it is complex, and – this should come as no surprise – that such cells are very sensitive to the effects of light.

For the immune system to prepare antibodies to attack an infection or other threat, it first has to recognise the invader and produce a line of T-cells which are specific for it. These are the white cells which are attacked by the AIDS virus. In the course of their development, they can either become T-helpers, which stimulate the immune system to attack a suspected threat, or T-suppressors, which subdue that attack. The key measure which is used by immunologists is the helper/suppressor ratio. This may be high in allergies and in acute infections, when the body is trying to mobilise the immune system to fight what it sees as an attack. A low ratio and therefore too many suppressors can cause lowered resistance to infection, and even to cancer. In AIDS the ratio is often very low, as the T-helpers are killed off by the virus more rapidly than the T-suppressors.

Formal introductions

Before either T-helpers or suppressors can be produced in response to an antigen, such as infecting organisms or potentially allergic foods or inhalants, the antigen has to be introduced to them. This very British transaction is performed by a category of cells known as antigen presenting, or AP cells.

The skin contains two different types of AP cells. The first type, the Langerhans cell, stimulates the production of T-helpers.[1] The Granstein cell, on the other hand, leads to the production of T-suppressor cells.[2] Both types appear to be killed – or at least have their effect blocked – by ultraviolet.[3] The Langerhans are more sensitive than the Granstein cells, so a low dose of UVB can probably reduce the immune response.

However, this refers to studies that were done on narrow-waveband light, and the maximum effect appears to be at around 297 nanometres. Since this is almost exactly the cut-off point for radiation reaching the earth's surface (the rest is filtered out by ozone in the atmosphere), there seems to be little or no risk of a damaging effect from ordinary sunlight, even on tropical mountains, in broad midday sunlight, in summer.

Light nourishes the immune system

On the other hand, there is another category of cell in the skin called keratinocytes. These do not present antigens, but they do appear to produce a chemical known as interleukin-1 or IL-1.[4] The name is unimportant, since it has been known by at least half a dozen other names in the time that we have been aware of it. What is important is the effect; it stimulates T-cells to reproduce and increase in number.

In contrast to the relatively slow process of antigen presentation, the development of new antibodies and of a viable immune response, which may take up to a fortnight, the response to interleukin-1 takes only a few hours.[5] It mobilises the immune response to all sorts of external factors. We now know that although exposure to monochromatic (narrow-waveband) ultraviolet light may kill off the cells that produce this chemical, broad-spectrum light, even simply the full waveband of ultraviolet light, appears to stimulate its production.[6]

Since the experiments that show suppression were done with light of 270 NM, which is *never* obtained naturally from sunlight, we probably need have no fear of sunlight damaging our immune system at all. But we can make use of the stimulating, IL-1-producing effect of light to assist our immune systems in keeping us well.

This response to sunlight probably explains the observation by Dr Frick in 1974 that exposure to ultraviolet light raises the number of white cells in the blood, increases the ability to deal with infections and improves general health.[7] This is backed up by some Russian studies which found that the ability of white cells to deal with infections is approximately doubled by ultraviolet light.[8] They now use this in schools and factories, and naturally in their long dark winters it is able to show a substantial reduction in health problems.

The only opportunity that we in the UK have to look at sunlight deprivation of similar severity is in the case of scientists on the Arctic and Antarctic standing bases operated by all the major powers. It is a recognised fact that men returning from expeditions or tours of duty on the polar ice-caps, where sunlight is in short supply at times, develop upper respiratory infections in large numbers on reentering 'civilisation'. Studies on their blood show that their white-cell counts go down substantially during the arctic winter.

Keeping the balance

Since so much immune function seems to originate in the skin, and since vitamin D is also manufactured in the skin, it is interesting to speculate whether there is a connection. The evidence in this direction is a tease: it raises the interest, but gives nothing tangible. In 1984 a study in Japan looked at T-helper and T-suppressor levels in osteoporosis, the bone-loss disease associated with ageing. The researchers reasoned that osteoporosis is likely to be an immune dysfunction, since it occurs with ageing – as do many immune problems; it occurs in rheumatoid arthritis, which is known to be an immune disorder; and it is more common in women, particularly around the time of childbirth and after the menopause. They found that the ratio of helper to suppressor cells was fifty per cent higher in osteoporotic patients.[9]

They then gave these patients vitamin D for two months, and found that this brought down the T-helper/suppressor ratio in every case to around the normal. In people of the same age without osteoporosis, who had a normal T-helper/T-suppressor ratio to start with, vitamin D does not alter this. It seems then that vitamin D brings raised T-helper/suppressor ratios back to normal, and reduces the allergic tendency that results from them.

Since ultraviolet light also has an effect on the immune cells in the skin, both regulating the ratio and increasing the total number of white cells, we are left wondering just how important an immune regulator vitamin D may be, and how dependent we are on sunlight for a smoothly functioning immune system. It stimulates the immune response, but at the same time provides the means for controlling and regulating that response. Without it, it seems, we run a much greater risk of a disordered immune system. With it, we can keep our immunity running like a well-tuned engine.

CHAPTER 11

See me, tan me, touch me, heal me

The skin is the largest organ of your body. Far from being a simple envelope without which your body would fall apart the skin has many functions, we have come to appreciate over recent years.

Any single-celled organism, such as an amoeba, is surrounded by a cell wall or membrane. This enables it to maintain the difference between the environment inside and that outside itself. It cannot do this simply by excluding the outside world; this would starve the cell to death. The membrane must both identify components of the outside environment, determining for example whether or not they are food, and control the selective admission into the cell of those chemicals that it needs. Clearly this process is crucial to the health and success of any organism, large or small.

A living frontier

All our needs, apart from that for food, are identified and fulfilled through our skin and our sensory organs. These organs are specialised derivatives of skin. The eyes, the nose, even the brain itself, are derived from primitive dermal tissue. Starting, in the early foetal stages, as simply the outermost layer of the body, dermal tissue develops into a complex set of systems for interacting with the environment.

The skin can perform 4 basic functions – it can sense, defend, express and ingest.

The *sense* function of the skin is performed by the nerve endings which detect touch, pain and pleasure. They enable us, even without using the special sense organs such as the eyes, to detect whether an environment is friendly or hostile to us. They even enable us, by contact with another person, to detect through their muscle tone, the quality of their touch, and the electrical charge and resistance of their skin, much of the nature of their feelings towards us. It is easy to lie down the telephone, but who can lie in a kiss?

As well as detecting pain and advising withdrawal from the painful stimulus, the skin also has inbuilt *defences* against a range of damaging environmental factors. Mechanical and chemical agents are excluded by the resilient, elastic underlying structure of the collagen in the dermis, as well as by the layer of dead cells that makes up the epidermis. This also presents an intact barrier against micro-organisms, as do the oils that are secreted on to the surface of our skin, when they are activated by ultraviolet light.[1] UV itself gets no further than the skin, but only a small proportion of it is reflected; much of it is transmitted into the epidermis and dermis, where it can have very definite effects on the skin, and then on the body in general.[2] The skin protects itself from excessive ultraviolet by producing melanin, which blocks the radiation effectively, but it only produces sufficient melanin to limit UV light, not to exclude it entirely.[3]

We *express* ourselves through our skin in a variety of ways. The skin is very important to doctors, as it is the easiest and readiest source of information about the body within. Nowadays we have sophisticated methods of 'seeing' the inside of the body, such as the CAT scan, but good medicine has always depended and still does depend on a careful physical examination of the patient, which is in large part an examinination of the patient's skin. Some diseases of the whole body are fairly obvious on the skin, such as anaemia, jaundice and extreme exhaustion; others require a specialised eye. In the five-element system of traditional Chinese medicine, for example, important diagnostic clues can be obtained from skilled interpretation of skin colour.

The other important signal that the skin gives is through smell, and this includes chemicals known as pheromone which can transmit sexual and emotional signals without either sender or recipient being consciously aware of them. When we kiss, as well as enjoying the touch sensation, we exchange pheromone signals.

Skin repair kit

All of these functions depend on a healthy skin, and healthy skin requires to be fed regularly. What it *ingests*, apart from the nutrients that are transmitted to it in the blood, is sunlight. The skin and eyes are the only organs capable of absorbing sunlight, and they do so voraciously, with effects that involve the whole body. The skin itself requires an adequate intake of sunlight in order to stay healthy. There is a long list of skin diseases which are benefited by sunlight and particularly by ultraviolet light. Possibly the best known of these is psoriasis, which affects about three per cent of the population.

Sufferers develop red scaly plaques of thickened skin, particularly over areas where there is friction, such as elbows and knees, but sometimes over the whole body. The top layer of the skin, the dead cells of the stratum corneum, is much thicker, and flakes off easily because the next layer down is less developed, causing poor attachment of the stratum corneum. As a result of this thickening, the skin is much more reflective to ultraviolet light.[4] In fact, simple exposure of the skin to ultraviolet may benefit the disease, but it is made much more effective if the transmission can be improved by application of an oily lubricant, such as vaseline, before ultraviolet treatment. This technique has cleared ninety per cent of patients, although it takes a lot of treatments.[5]

A substantial business has built up around the treatment of psoriasis, particularly in Israel, where the shores of the Dead Sea seem to be areas with a particularly beneficial effect. Like Death Valley in California, this is one of the hottest and most barren places on earth, and is also below sea level. The climate in such places appears to produce a self-sustaining hole in the surrounding weather, through which the sun shines intensely hour after hour.

It seems likely that this is why the Dead Sea benefits psoriasis. However, we now know that the effect can be greatly enhanced by giving the patients substances which sensitise them to ultraviolet effects. Essentially these substances are dyes which attach to molecules within the body and enable them to absorb light radiation more effectively, thus increasing the impact of sunlight.[6] Because of their proven effects in psoriasis, the major group is known as psoralens.

Surprisingly, the treatment of acne with sunlight or ultraviolet has been much less studied. There have been no controlled scientific studies to prove that it works. However, anybody who has suffered from acne – and this includes most of us at one time or another in our lives – will have noticed that sunlight does make a difference. There are a number of reasons why this should be so. If acne is caused or made worse by bacteria in the skin, as many scientists believe, then ultraviolet light will help to kill the bacteria. On the other hand, it will also stimulate our immune response to these bacteria, and this would fit with the observed fact that acne often gets slightly worse immediately after sunlight exposure. From being unable to handle the bacteria effectively and remove them from the skin, we suddenly go into the attack and clear them out of the skin by the only route available – through spots.

If a build-up of dead skin cells and cell debris clogs the pores of the sebaceous glands and causes a back pressure and swelling of the gland which then gets infected, ultraviolet light will increase the turnover of cells and help to clear this blockage. Whichever way it works, light therapy is a far more attractive prospect in acne than long-term low-dose antibiotics, which can cause allergies, often interfere with the organisms in the bowel and do not work very well anyway.

Another disease of the skin which improves on sunlight therapy is vitiligo, in which patches of white, depigmented skin appear for no clear reason. It has been suggested that this is associated with vitamin B12 deficiency, but nevertheless treatment with sunlight combined with psoralens has a mildly beneficial effect in at least seventy per cent of cases.[7] Even more effective, according to a recent study, is a combination of the amino-acid phenylalanine with regular sunlight exposure.[8]

Improvement is slow, as the pigmentation takes time to develop; but when it does reappear it is long lasting. The same psoralen/UV light treatment benefits an unpleasant malignant disease of the skin called mycosis fungoides, as it also does urticaria, or nettle rash, even if this is triggered by sunlight itself.[9] Nobody knows how the treatment works in this case, but work it does.

Natural healing

One skin effect that is easy to explain is the benefit to wound and ulcer healing, particularly if these occur in areas of poor circulation. Clearly, sunlight increases the blood flow through the area and therefore the supply of nutrients to the injury. Even more important may be the effect of biological radiation. All the studies on ultraviolet radiation of and from living cells has shown that trauma is a very effective way of stimulating a cell to radiate.[10] This, of course, may go a long way to explaining why inserting a needle into an acupuncture point in the skin can stimulate bioenergetic responses throughout the body.

It also explains why a skin wound bioradiates strongly for two or three days. This radiation stimulates cell growth and division at the edges of the wound, leading to more rapid healing. Irradiation of the cells from outside with ultraviolet light also stimulates them to radiate in turn, and this will enhance healing too. It is clear, once again, that sunlight is woven into the fabric of our lives. It is not just useful in wound healing, it is an essential nutrient for the skin.

Sunlight – essential to a balanced diet

Perhaps more fascinating still are the effects that the skin has on the rest of the body. There are several of these in which sunlight clearly plays a part. The first, and the best known, is the production of vitamin D. This requires sunlight for its manufacture from the precursor of cholesterol. When released through the body and activated, vitamin D improves our efficiency in the metabolism of minerals such as calcium and magnesium, and also of protein. A Russian study found that vitamin D produces a thirty per cent improvement in our conservation of protein.[11]

Interleukin-1 is a newly discovered molecule that is produced by the most superficial cells in the skin, keratinocytes. It stimulates white cells to multiply and is a vital stage in the mobilising of an immune response to any infection. This may explain the observation that gamma globulins (the proteins in the blood which contain antibodies) are increased for a month after exposure to ultraviolet light. It also makes sense of the observation that polar explorers suffer frequent infections on return to civilisation. In fact, the Russians refer to 'light-hunger, a disease for the far North and polar regions,' which involves a general weakening of the body's defences against infection and chronic illnesses of all sorts.

The skin also comprises an enormous bed of capillary blood vessels, through which the blood circulates, and in which it can be exposed to sunlight. It is the red blood cells in these capillaries that give the pink colour to our skins. When skin goes red from sunburn or after being smacked, for instance, this is caused by these capillaries dilating to allow more blood into them.

The experience of American physicians working with the Knott technique showed that ultraviolet irradiation of the blood had some very powerful effects on the system at large. But the structure of the skin makes it a highly efficient organ for irradiating the blood with sunlight. The cells of the blood which have been gently bathed in ultraviolet light by this method are stimulated to produce their own ultraviolet radiation, and they carry this effect in the circulation to every cell in the body. This provides the light energy necessary to fuel our essential chemical reactions.

Now that the evidence is starting to mount again in favour of ultraviolet light for a variety of health problems, many of us are going to want to take advantage of its effects. It would be

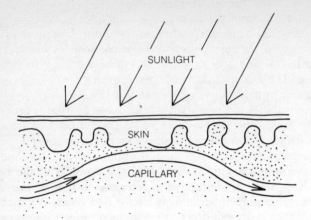

nice to imagine that the government will provide a 'photarium' in every small community, but few things on earth can be less likely. We shall all have to make our own arrangements for regular trips to the sun, full-spectrum lighting or some more specific form of light therapy.

CHAPTER 12
The solar-powered athlete

For forty years we have been missing out on a literally golden opportunity to become healthier. Whether we are rundown office workers or athletes in training, the effects of ultraviolet light on fitness are considerable. One example is the improvement in the power, endurance and recovery time of muscles – and this includes the heart muscle. Fitness training undertaken in sunlight or with exposure to ultraviolet light is far more effective than without it.

When the skin is exposed to sunlight, the blood passing through it receives ultraviolet and other radiation. The effect is a gentler version of that achieved with the Knott technique, in which blood is removed, irradiated with ultraviolet and reinjected. The capacity of the blood to carry oxygen goes up, and this happens within an hour and lasts for several weeks. This means that less work is demanded of the heart. At the same time the amount of oxygen being supplied to the tissues, including the tissue of the heart itself, increases. In some studies the oxygen-carrying capacity went up as much as fifty per cent.[1] This irradiation of blood cells also stimulates them to produce their own bioradiation. They then pass through the whole of the body, transmitting these impulses to all the other cells.

Protti in Milan, and other researchers throughout Europe, found in the thirties that the radiation detectable from blood increased after food, and decreased with fatigue.[2] After a day's work or several hours physical exertion it was down to almost nothing. In a couple of hours it had returned nearly to normal. Inhaling oxygen had a boosting effect on bioradiation, but only for about one hour. The effect of ultraviolet exposure, on the other hand, lasted for hours or even days.[3] In other words, when fuelled with ultraviolet light energy, the blood becomes a living battery, supplying energy to the working muscles and nerves.

The muscles underlying an area exposed directly to sunlight also show some local effects. There is an increase in the amount of blood flowing through the muscles, as the blood vessels relax, together with a measurable rise in the temperature of the muscle.[4] At the same time the work capacity and endurance of the muscle goes up. After a single dose of UV, the effect lasts for at least five days. Whereas the increase in oxygen capacity of the blood is a general effect – and treating, say, one arm will affect the whole body – the increase of blood flow through the muscles is a local effect, and only operates in muscles under the area exposed to UV.

Today's athletes can learn from the past

The Greeks obviously appreciated some of the importance of sunlight; their athletes trained naked out of doors, thus exposing all their muscles to its beneficial effect. I fear that as a fitness aid this would have been less well received at the last Commonwealth Games in Edinburgh than it evidently was in Ancient Greece. But there is no reason why gymnasiums and health clubs should not be equipped with full-spectrum lighting, enabling athletes and customers to train in ultraviolet light. It would not be necessary to train naked, but is seems that one might be well advised to avoid synthetic fabrics where possible. Natural fibres appear to be much better transmitters of ultraviolet light than synthetics, as well as being generally drier and more absorbent.[5] The heavier the fabric, and the stronger the dyes in it, the more it filters out UV.

Because of the blood's increased oxygen-carrying capacity, athletes would find that their respiratory rate also decreased, their lungs would not need to work so hard. By the same token, their resting heart rate would go down, and the amount by which their heart rate went up after exercise would be less.

When a group of generally unfit students at the University of Illinois was treated with ultraviolet light as well as physical

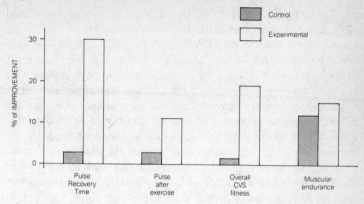

education classes, their pulse rate after exercise came down by more than ten points on average. The students who did the same exercise but did not receive the UV light only had a three point improvement. The experimental group also found that their recovery time after exercise went down by thirty per cent, and their overall muscular fitness improved by half as much again as did that of the control group.

But the really startling results of this study were in the cardio-vascular fitness tests, where the experimental group improved by almost 20 per cent, compared to a minute 1.5 per cent improvement in the control group. Cardiovascular fitness, in this case, referred to a combined measure of a number of different parameters, such as resting pulse, rise of pulse after exertion, blood pressure lying and standing, rise in blood pressure after exertion, and time for pulse rate to return to normal after exertion. The students also reported an increase in their interest and enthusiasm for classwork, and those receiving ultraviolet developed only half the number of colds that the control group suffered.[6]

Fuel reserves

People training in such an environment would also experience an increase in the amount of glycogen in their muscles and in the liver. Carbohydrates in the diet are broken down into molecules of sugar, which either circulate as blood sugar and are therefore readily available but also readily lost, or else they are stored for later use as glycogen. Glycogen molecules consist of thousands of glucose or sugar units joined together in numbers of small clusters. Each cluster contains thirty four molecules of glucose. It represents the main source of energy for normal physical exertion, and is the limiting factor for endurance. When all the available glycogen in muscle is used up, the muscle relies on what energy can be brought to it in the blood. One of the most important effects of physical training is to increase the store of glycogen in the muscle, and this explains why athletes normally do not train for two or three days before a competitive event – it takes this long for the glycogen store in the muscles to be built up again.

When human subjects are exposed to UV, the glycogen level in their tissues dives in the first hour or so, and then the enzymes which manufacture glycogen are stimulated. The level of glycogen stored in the tissues rises steadily for about sixteen hours. Because of this timing, ultraviolet light or sunlight in the one or two days preceding a competition would appear to be ideal. Clearly, also, athletes who train in or come from tropical countries have a head start on those of us who inhabit these grey islands.[7]

In parallel with the increase in glycogen stores goes a decrease in blood sugar – or, more precisely, a normalisation of abnormal blood sugar. Although most cells in the body do not depend on glucose, being able to use their glycogen stores, the one tissue that is most dependent on blood glucose, and which uses up twenty per cent of it, is the brain. As a result, the way we feel depends very much on the circulating level of glucose. When the blood sugar is high, we are likely to feel alert, clear-headed, energetic and generally capable; if it gets too high we may even feel tense, twitchy, anxious and agitated. It is precisely this range of effects that we develop after a cup of strong tea or coffee, and it is largely through raising the blood sugar that these 'social poisons' work.

When the blood sugar goes down we tend to find ourselves running out of energy and becoming drowsy, irritable and emotional. It is then that our inbuilt weaknesses show through, such as migraines, fainting, hallucinations, attacks of crying or tantrums, or simply falling asleep at the job. When the blood sugar is up it is anxiety and anger symptoms that prevail; when it is down we experience the depression and exhaustion. This may explain why so many of us can be hell to live with at times; when our blood sugar is up we pick a fight with somebody, but when it drops we suddenly find outselves slumping and wondering why everybody hates us. Many women find that the problem of hypoglycaemia – low blood sugar – is much worse before their period.[8,9].

The effect of light on blood sugar is quite remarkable, and depends on the wavelength or colour of light used. The graph shows the blood-sugar level of rabbits during constant exposure to light of different colours. Blue and green lights do not make a great deal of difference, red causes it to go up rapidly and ultraviolet reduces it.

This effect was further confirmed in human studies when it

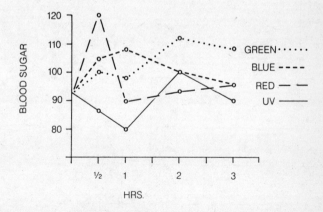

was shown that the blood sugar of diabetics was also lowered by ultraviolet. Diabetics do not produce enough insulin, the molecule that lowers blood sugar by assisting ths sugar into cells. Their blood sugar is therefore unstable, and they commonly have to take injections of insulin to help to bring it down. Pincussen showed that by using daily doses of UV light, he could bring the blood sugar of diabetics down very effectively. There was an immediate improvement after the first day of treatment, and over a period of up to a fortnight the blood sugar slowly settled down to normal and stayed there. It showed no signs of decreasing to below the normal level, so there is no reason for us to think that UV has a harmful hypoglycaemic effect.[10]

Not all of us need our blood sugar lowering drastically, and it appears that a ratio of ten per cent ultraviolet, ninety per cent visible light produces the best stablising effect in normal people, as well as having the best result in raising glycogen stores in liver and muscle. This proportion, you will not be amazed to hear, is close to that found in natural sunlight, and is the balance aimed at by modern full-spectrum light fixtures.

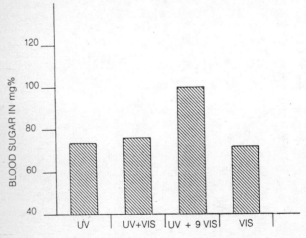

EFFECT OF DIFFERENT COMPOSITIONS OF LIGHT ON BLOOD SUGAR

Sunlight adjusts the gauge

An interesting angle on the connection between light and fitness comes from the finding that the pineal gland, the famous third eye, regulates our whole hormonal balance. It is now clear that the pineal produces melatonin in response to darkness. The effect of this chemical is to make you drowsy and more able to sleep, and also slower at simple tasks. But it appears that the pineal also regulates the output of the pituitary gland. This small gland at the base of the brain produces hormones that control the functioning of all the other endocrine glands, and thereby of every cell in the body.

Pituitary products include a thyroid-stimulating hormone (TSH), an adrenal-stimulating, or adrenocorticotrophic hormone (ACTH), and several other hormones with effects on the sexual glands in particular. With all of the endocrine functions, it is not a matter of 'if a little is good for you, then a lot will be better'. We need a precise balance of hormones in order to stay well, and an excess can be just as damaging as a deficiency. The thyroid gland, as we shall see later, can be overactive, leading to thyrotoxicosis; or underactive, causing myxoedema or hypothyroidism.

Proof of this comes from the work of Hollwich in 1980.[11] He studied the levels of ACTH, the adrenal-stimulating hormone, in the blood under natural and artificial light. After a fortnight in light from 'cool white' fluorescent tubes his subjects' ACTH levels had climbed to abnormally high, stress levels. Two weeks under daylight returned them to normal. But when the lights used were of a full-spectrum type, there was no significant increase in ACTH levels. In both cases, the light intensity was high – high enough, at 3500 lux, to suppress melatonin. So this was not a straightforward pineal effect of the type we can now easily recognise, but another mechanism altogether. As yet, we do not know how it operates, but the implication is that artificial light which is different in spectrum from sunlight puts a stress on the body, even over a period as short as two weeks, which is enough to persuade the pituitary to overproduce hormones.

One of the established methods of testing pituitary function is by the degree of response to insulin. Although insulin is required for keeping blood sugar down, it is normally counter-balanced and held in check by several other hormones within the body, and in particular by ACTH from the pituitary. If pituitary function is low, then the body cannot handle insulin properly and it will send the blood sugar down dramatically. If, on the other hand, the pituitary is overactive, there will be a generally high blood sugar. This is known to be a risk factor for hardening of the arteries, heart attacks and strokes. It also makes us more prone to infections. All of these are problems encountered by diabetics, who cannot produce enough insulin for themselves.

Sunlight entering the eyes prevents the pineal from inhibiting the pituitary, and thereby provides a counterbalance to the hypoglycaemic effect of sunlight hitting the skin.[12] Vitamin D and calcium also appear to have a stimulating effect on insulin,[13] and they are affected by UV light as well.

Insulin is also important as the molecule that conducts a wide range of nutrients, not just sugar, across the cell walls and into the cells. Without it there may be problems of cellular nutrition, even though the diet is adequate. But some athletes face the problem of finding time to get enough calories into their stomachs, not to mention all the other essential nutrients. Because they may be expending anything up to three times as much energy as the rest of us, they need to eat proportionately more.

Yet for every ounce they eat, they need also to take in the vitamins and minerals required for processing those calories into energy. To a nutritionally oriented physician, many of the recurrent health problems of athletes these days are strongly suggestive of a borderline nutritional state. In my own practice, I have certainly found that athletes in training may need to eat considerably more vitamins and minerals than the average person, just to prevent a deficiency.

There are several ways that sunlight can help this state of affairs. Firstly, by stimulating all of the hormonal system and metabolism it can increase the efficiency with which we use nutrients. Secondly, by enhancing insulin production it enables us to transport nutrients into our cells more effectively. Thirdly, an increase in vitamin D production will lead to an increase in our body's uptake of calcium, magnesium and protein from the diet. Magnesium deficiency has been found in athletes quite often, and supplementation can lead to an improvement in health generally as well as in sporting performance.[14]

Finally, joint problems and stress fractures are by no means rare in top athletes, and improved calcium and magnesium metabolism, with increased bone density, will unquestionably benefit this. As an example, bone density in Polynesian women has been found to be twenty per cent higher than in European woman of the same age.[15] Polynesians are not noted for their adherence to health foods, and communities have been known to survive for months on fish, coconuts, palm wine and little else – no salads or wholegrains at all. But they do live in the sun.

The role of the pineal in fitness now starts to look a little complex. Clearly, sunlight-induced suppression of melatonin will lead to a pituitary stimulus, increasing the output of all the hormonal glands. The next gland we should look at is the thyroid. Thyroid hormones are important in controlling the basal metabolic rate of the whole body – the rate at which cells burn up calories to produce energy and heat. A simple test of thyroid function is the basal temperature. The temperature is taken in the armpit for three minutes mimimum, first thing in the morning, before getting out of bed and before any activity at all. The ideal temperature is about 98.0°F, one that is below 97.5°F raises the possibility of a thyroid problem.

Symptoms of a thyroid deficiency commonly include depression, lack of energy, weight increase, cold sensitivity, excessive sleeping and a generally run-down system.[16] Sunlight, via the pineal-pituitary axis, stimulates the thyroid and benefits such problems. It also increases energy levels in general, together with resistance to disease, and the ability to burn up calories and lose weight. At the same time, the adrenal gland is stimulated in exactly the same fashion, with a consequent increase in the ability to handle stress, including physical stress. Muscular development is enhanced, and we feel better while we become fitter.

It comes as no surprise, though, that we need our beauty sleep. We need a period during the twenty four hours when the pineal *is* producing melatonin, and our metabolism is more or less shut down for repairs. It is known that adrenal steroid levels vary throughout the twenty four hours, climbing steadily through the day and dropping down at night. This shifts our metabolism from an outward-looking, active phase to a rest and recovery phase. The list of measures which vary throughout the day/night cycle is immense, ranging from rate of cell division to sensitivity to pain.

But this rhythm of sleeping and waking is controlled through the pineal, and needs both the light and the dark for a proper cycle. Nowadays, living indoors, we see very little of the necessary intensity of light. Are we spending less of our time either fully waking or sleeping, and more of it half awake? One of the components of ageing is a disorganisation of this cycle, with loss of the rhythmic alternation, leading to disturbed sleep patterns and to loss of the ability of our bodies to repair themselves. Interestingly, administration of pineal extract to rats increased their life-span by up to twenty five per cent.[17]

Even weight control can be assisted by attention to the pineal. The link-up here is through a substance called brown fat. Only discovered a few years ago, this is very different from ordinary fat. It appears to have a much higher turnover of calories and production of energy, and is a major heat source for the body. It also helps in reducing weight by using up calories. Unfortunately for many of us, our amount and activity of brown fat seems to be proportional to the calories we eat. The higher our calorie intake, the more brown fat activity, and so the more calories we burn off. But fasting or dieting gives our bodies the signal that we are in a period of hardship and energy should be conserved. So our brown fat activity decreases.

In several different species of mammals, it has been shown that melatonin given by mouth, or long nights leading to increased production of melatonin, can produce an increase in the amount of brown fat.[18] This melatonin-induced increase in brown fat leads inevitably to rise in the metabolic rate, which is helpful in controlling weight problems. Since diet won't do it, and since there is no wonder drug yet to trigger brown fat activity, the only way seems to be with melatonin. Once again, it appears that we need the down side and the up; we have to maintain a genuine rhythm of day and night in order to control our own health.

Regular exposure to sunlight, then, or to indoor lighting that includes the full spectrum of visible and ultraviolet light, can help us to get fitter, and to look and feel better. All the crucial biological signals dependent on sunlight hitting the skin are activated and sent to the rest of the body. Fitness in general and cardiovascular fitness in particular improve. We are able to build healthier muscles with greater endurance, to use up more calories more efficiently and to burn off fat deposits. All of these changes enable us to feel and look better. After all, nothing improves the appearance and texture of our skin more than a gentle tan. And nothing enhances our attractiveness so much as glowing healthy skin and a slim figure.

CHAPTER 13

The sun and the heart

Why is it that shift workers get more than twice as much heart diesease as the rest of us?[1] Is it because they smoke more or take less physical exercise outside work, or suffer more stress? Or is it because they are light-deficient? When a group in New Jersey looked at the life expectancy of hamsters with an inherited tendency towards heart attacks, they found that keeping them in constant light made them live twenty five per cent longer.[2] This result was obtained despite the fact that the longer-lived hamsters had had time to develop worse heart disease, according to anatomical measures. If, just supposing, we could carry this effect over to humans, the average life expectancy for men would be approximately ninety, with far more centenarians surviving.

Sunlight clears the channels

At the moment this study is a puzzle. We have no clear explanation for it, but there are a number of possibilities. For example, we do know that sunlight lowers cholesterol levels. Exposing human skin to sunlight for a couple of hours lowers the level of cholesterol in the skin by at least a half.[3] The effect is less in negro skin, suggesting that it is the ultraviolet, which melanin pigmentation filters out, that is causing the effect. It is also known that sunlight lowers the level of cholesterol in the blood stream in humans by 9 or 10 per cent.

We know that the reduction is greater the higher the starting cholesterol level; people with low or normal cholesterol to begin with are much less likely to see a significant drop than those with a raised cholesterol.[4] We also know that ultraviolet irradiation of foods can lower their cholesterol content.[5] In some cases, too, simple sunbathing can bring a raised level of fats (known as triglycerides) down.[6]

The difficult question to answer in all of this is just how important cholesterol is in the development of heart disease. We know that a raised cholesterol is associated with a greater risk of heart disease, but this does not necessarily mean that cholesterol causes heart disease. An increase in the number of tourists is normally associated with summer, but it may not be causing summer. The summer may be causing tourists to breed rapidly, or on the other hand they may all just turn up together in summer by coincidence!

It is true that cholesterol is a fat-soluble substance, and an increase in the fat content of blood is often associated with an increase in cholesterol. Cholesterol also precipitates out of blood on to and into the lining of arteries, and forms the plaque which clogs them up and leads to blockages or thromboses. A rise in the circulating level of calcium in the blood can play a part in this; the bulk of the calcium in our bodies should be in our bones, and we require vitamin D in order to place it there and keep it there.

It was, until recently, thought that once a cholesterol plaque formed in a blood vessel, it was quite immovable. We now know that this is untrue. There is a simple technique called chelation, which is viewed without enthusiasm by the orthodox medical profession, despite a very large number of research papers describing and measuring it.[7] Chelation involves using a chemical called EDTA, which combines very strongly with minerals in the blood and is then excreted along with those minerals. It clears all the toxic and unwanted minerals out of the body, together with the essential ones – but the essential ones can be replaced at the same time so that the patient does not run short of them at all. The method leads in some cases to a dramatic drop in blood cholesterol and a declogging of the arteries with removal or at least diminution of the plaque.[8]

Sunlight can lower cholesterol dramatically and produce the same effect as chelation. It can also protect against the development of coronary artery disease and the other forms of hardening of the arteries in the first place.[9] This might well be why shift workers suffer from more heart disease than the rest of us, and may also explain the observation that heart disease is more common the further we go from the equator. In fact, heart disease and cancer do tend to go together to some extent; areas and groups with a high cancer risk tend to have a high risk of heart disease also. In chapter 6 we saw the effect of latitude on cancer; there is about 2.5 times as much cancer in northern climates as there is near to the equator. This parallels the incidence of heart disease.

The other common misconception about cholesterol is to see it entirely as a baddie. This is desperately wrong. Cholesterol is the precursor of our entire catalogue of steroid hormones. Without cholesterol we would have no hormones and therefore no sex, no ability to respond to stress and no ability to reproduce. Although it has not been shown that sunlight causes cholesterol to be converted into steroid hormones, we do know that cholesterol is lowered and sex hormones are raised by sunlight and ultraviolet light exposure.

The mellow mineral

Another factor which plays a major part in heart disease is magnesium. This is one of the most abundant minerals inside our cells, and is important in an enormous range of functions. A deficiency of magnesium can lead to psychiatric symptoms such as anxiety, insomnia, fatigue and irritability, as well as premenstrual syndrome, disorders of calcium metabolism including osteoporosis or thinning of the bones, and also to heart disease.[10]

There are a great number of enzymes which depend on magnesium for their operation, but the single most important one is probably the 'pump' which controls the flow of minerals across the cell wall from the serum and extracellular fluid, into the cell itself.[11] Cells without enough magnesium around tend to be oversensitive and irritable, firing off at slight provocation, just like a pre-menstrual woman (sexist remark). If nerve cells do this, it may cause a sustained discharge rather than a regular, rhythmic one. This is why the typical symptoms of magnesium deficiency are a tendency to muscle cramps, spasms, sensitivity to noises and other external stimuli, as well as a tendency to irregular heart rhythm, and to spasm of the coronary arteries leading in extreme cases to heart attack. Giving magnesium intravenously after a heart attack, saves lives, by preventing the heart from going into arrhythmia.[12]

Magnesium deficiency can also lead to high blood pressure, high cholesterol and fat levels in the blood, and thromboses.[13] So magnesium is essential for health, and particularly for cardiac health. It is also the crucial trace element in the chlorophyll of green plants. Just as iron is necessary to hold the haemoglobin molecule of human blood into shape, so magnesium provides the shaping force for chlorophyll. The best source available for magnesium, therefore, is green leafy plants. It also occurs in reasonable quantities in nuts and in dairy products, but in milk in particular it is heavily outbalanced by calcium.

Calcium and magnesium have related, complementary roles in the cells of our body, rather like the accelerator and the brake on a car. Both are necessary in reasonable degree, and without a proper balance between the two, things can go seriously awry. Unfortunately, it seems that the human body has spent most of its evolutionary time in an environment which is rich in magnesium, but not so rich in calcium. This would be the case if we had evolved eating plants and vegetables, which in prehistorical times were presumably there for the taking, but had not started milking cows or other domestic animals until much later on.

The consequence is that we have a much better developed mechanism for conserving calcium than for conserving magnesium.[14] The effect of vitamin D, for example, on calcium balance is quite clear cut. It influences every mechanism of calcium intake and output to ensure that calcium is conserved, and it can make a difference of 2.5 times in the percentage of calcium that we absorb from our food.[15] With magnesium, on the other hand, the picture is more complex. Vitamin D increases the absorption of magnesium from our diet, and in vitamin D deficiency we need more magnesium; but an excessive intake of vitamin D causes greater loss of magnesium in the urine, and again increases the requirement [16,17]. We need to get our vitamin D levels just right, in order to make the most of the limited amount of magnesium available to us.

In laboratory studies, the signs of an experimental magnesium deficiency are very similar to those of experimental vitamin D toxicity.[18]

- Hardening of the coronary arteries
- Calcification of the arterial wall
- Necrosis of the heart muscle
- Raised blood-fat levels

Protection against the toxic effects of excessive vitamin D appears to be possible by greatly increasing the magnesium intake; but beneficial as it may be, not many of us would elect to live constantly on large volumes of salad. It makes more sense to avoid a high vitamin D intake rather than to have to treat it.

The British complaint

In Britain, food is not supplemented with vitamin D to anywhere near the extent that it is in the USA. As a result, vitamin D deficiency is much more common, especially in winter. This is no more desirable than a vitamin D excess. The only sensible approach is to obtain adequate amounts of sunlight and manufacture our vitamin D as it is meant to be done, through a system that has inbuilt checks and balances; an overdose of vitamin D from sunlight has never been recorded.

Magnesium is also essential for the regulation of blood sugar levels.[19] In this it complements the direct effect of sunlight on blood sugar. As discussed in chapter 12, all frequencies of light have different effects on our blood sugar. Red light causes it to go up most, and blue and ultraviolet light cause it to go down. The best combination of frequencies for regulating blood sugar correctly appears to match the spectrum of sunlight. Since sunlight is the environment in which we evolved, this is hardly surprising.

There is no question that sugar is bad for the heart. As well as suppressing the ability of the body's white cells to fight off infection, sugar contributes to weight problems which put an added burden on the heart muscle. Simply eating refined sugar depletes us of essential minerals and vitamins that are needed for proper heart functioning, such as chromium and vitamin B6. It also appears that sugar itself causes or worsens atherosclerosis (hardening of the arteries). A high blood sugar level, such as that experienced by diabetics, is a definite risk factor for all the cardiovascular problems such as heart attack and angina.

Lighting the interior

Sunlight in general, and ultraviolet light in particular, appears to have powerful beneficial effects on the heart. Ultraviolet irradiation of the blood, whether in a clinical setting such as the Knott technique, or by irradiation as it circulates through the skin by means of sunbathing, can increase the oxygen-carrying capacity of the blood dramatically.[20] This means that the same amount of circulating blood can supply more oxygen for the tissues, including the heart muscle itself. Sunlight can also lower the blood-cholesterol level significantly – and by a greater amount the higher it is to start with.

The effect on blood pressure is even more striking. A single dose of sunlight can bring the blood pressure down immediately, and the effect takes two or three days to wear off.[21] Two doses of sunlight on consecutive days can keep the blood pressure down for over a week. The effect is, as with cholesterol, much more marked when the blood pressure is abnormally high to start with. One study found that in people with a normal starting blood pressure, the systolic pressure (the higher of the two numbers of blood pressure) was brought down by 6 mm, but in the hypertensives the average drop was 17 mm of mercury.

At the same time as the blood pressure came down, there was

a substantial increase in the output of the heart in the majority of patients. Since the pressure drop was associated with this increase in cardiac efficiency, it must be due at least in part to the known relaxation and widening of the blood vessels – and increase in blood flow through the large muscles of the body – that occur when we are exposed to sunlight.

In Cureton's study, conducted at the University of Illinois in 1945, cardiovascular fitness (based on measures such as the resting pulse rate, increase in pulse after exercise, lying and standing blood pressure, and so on) improved far more in students who received short doses of ultraviolet light before their training sessions. In the experimental group (receiving UV) the improvement was nearly 20 per cent, whereas the control group benefited only 1.5 per cent.[22] This effect was measured after three months, and other studies have shown that an improvement in physical fitness after sunlight lasts for weeks and months, rather than days.

Using sunlight or ultraviolet light to treat blood pressure and heart problems is safer, freer from side effects, more generally beneficial to the whole body and definitely more pleasant than having to take antihypertensive drugs. But in a world which spends 1.2 billion dollars a year on only on the top three blood pressure drugs, surely the use of sunlight is also more moral?

UV – the nourishing element

As well as the benefit to the heart itself, the consequences of sunlight therapy include improved perfusion (blood flow) to all the tissues of the body. For decades now, doctors in Russia have been using sunlight and ultraviolet light therapy on patients with arteriosclerosis.[23] They have found that as well as improving heart function, the blood supply to the brain can be improved, even in patients with arteriosclerosis of the brain.

Many victims of angina, hypertension and ischaemic heart disease feel lousy in general. They complain of headaches, dizziness, difficulty in thinking, chronic weakness and fatigue, lack of muscular strength or stamina. Much of this is due to poor blood supply to their tissues, with a consequent build-up of toxic metabolites. These include chemicals, such as lactic acid and ammonia, which are natural products of our metabolism, together with unmetabolised fats and toxic minerals. Methods such as chelation therapy unclog the arteries and help to clear these toxins out of the sytem. They would not be necessary if we had employed nature's own method of detoxification, which is the application of sunlight.

Once again, it is only the Russians who have fully appreciated this effect of sunlight and put it to use. Their experiments showed that animals exposed to the correct doses of sunlight were capable of clearing a wide range of toxins out of their system considerably quicker than animals reared away from the sun. The toxins that they studied included quartz and coal dusts, toxic minerals such as lead, cadmium and mercury, liver poisons such as carbon tetrachloride, and the neurotoxins which these days are so heavily used worldwide as insecticides. They found that sunlight speeded up the clearance of toxins from the body twice to as much as twenty times.[24] The best effect was obtained when sunlight exposure had started some time before exposure to the toxin.

Nowadays, some Russian miners are required to have a treatment with ultraviolet light every day when they leave the coal-face.[25] If we offered this treatment to our own coal-miners, they might not only suffer fewer ill effects from what is, after all, a very punishing occupation; they might be happier people all round!

As we shall see in the next chapter, sunlight also plays an important part in helping us to handle stress. This is a concept which it is easy to misunderstand. Many people say: 'I operate better under stress; I need a certain amount of it to get me going.' They are in fact talking about stimulation, which we all need regularly in a variety of forms in order to keep us functioning. This is not stress. Stress occurs when the incoming stimulus exceeds our ability to handle it, or we handle it only with damaging consequences to ourselves.

To use a physical example, we all know that exercise is good for us. A run or a workout on a regular basis can make us feel much better. But if we are forced to exercise violently, beyond our capacity, or to exercise when we are already exhausted, then our bodies are likely to suffer. This applies equally to our minds and our nervous system.

Features associated with chronic stress in humans include overweight, smoking and excessive intake of tea, coffee, alcohol, sugar and other generally non-nutritious foods. All of these factors are potentially damaging to the cardiovascular system; they increase the risk of heart and artery diseases. Raised blood pressure, poor peripheral circulation, angina and heart attacks have all been connected to stress. By its impact on the mind, stress can damage the body – and the heart is one of the main targets.

Sunlight has implications for all of these problems. It relaxes the muscles, unclogs the arteries and helps us to cope with life. It soothes the mind and heals the body. *It should be an essential part of any stress management programme, or any attempt by individuals or groups to return to health.*

CHAPTER 14

Sex – and sunlight

Nude sunbathing makes you sexier!

If you turned to this chapter first, I would not want the opening sentence to disappoint you, and in any case it's true. For a number of general reasons, exposure to sunlight is likely to make us feel healthier and improve our sex lives – but there are some very specific reasons also.

The general reasons include a lowering of blood pressure, an improvement in the flow of blood and a rise in the oxygen content of that blood, all of which will stimulate the metabolism within *all* the tissues of the body.[1] The brain is, without a doubt, the most important sexual organ; without it we would be unable to feel anything physical, emotional or spiritual for anybody else. Anything that improves the blood and oxygen supply to the brain – and sunlight does – can only improve our capacity for loving, both physically and emotionally.

Ultraviolet aphrodisiac

The warm, relaxed sense of wellbeing that we obtain from lying in the sun must be one of the closest things on earth to the warmth and security of snuggling up in our mother's arms. Such a feeling cannot be less than beneficial to a healthy sex life, but it seems to go deeper than this. Sunlight is, we now know, essential to health in a variety of ways. Along with protein, calories, vitamins, minerals and all the others, it is an essential nutrient. Sunbathing gives us something we need, particularly nowadays when most of us spend our whole lives indoors; it recharges our batteries. It replenishes our stores of the principal life force of this planet, and so we have more to give to others.

It is not for nothing that a caring person is referred to as warm, and an unfriendly or unloving one as cold.

Several years ago I worked in the Solomon Islands, in the Pacific Ocean, just south of the equator. It was regularly remarked upon there that most European couples arrived certain that they had filled their quota of 2.4 children, and never expected to have any more. But two years later many of them left bemusedly clutching a babe-in-arms. The local people said simply that the child was a 'gift belong Solomons'. We pale and sickly expatriates were probably no different from the post that, supposedly dead, is stuck into the ground to support a washing line, and sprouts roots and branches. This was another hazard of Solomon life! There is no doubt that the level of fertility is higher in tropical climates for all living things. Humans are not such an exception as they have always liked to think themselves.

Sunlight falling on the skin can raise the level of sex hormones in the blood. This effect has been known for over fifty years, and has been the basis of, for example, measures to improve the laying rate of hens.[2] But the same thing does happen in humans. When researchers gave doses of ultraviolet to subjects in Boston, USA, they found that a course of five doses, of increasing duration, each of them sufficient to produce slight reddening of the skin, could double the male hormone output.[3]

This ties in with the studies which have shown that levels of testosterone, the major male hormone, rise by about twenty per cent through the summer, reaching a peak in September.[4] In females, the effect was somewhat less but still measurable. The part of the body exposed to ultraviolet also made a difference. Some increase could be achieved whichever area of skin received the irradiation, but while exposing the back produced a doubling in hormones, exposing the skin of the genitals could cause the hormone level to triple.

At this dose level they also found that five treatments was the ideal number. The effect ceased increasing with further exposure. After this experiment, the rise in hormone levels took a fortnight or more to return to normal, and the beneficial impact on health, mental wellbeing and sexuality would of course take longer still to wear off. In other words, a week in the sun can make all the difference.

Naturally, the greater the amount of skin exposed to sunlight or ultraviolet, the larger the effect. Doubling the area of skin exposed will double the amount of UV we can absorb. It is tempting to reflect that the bikini-clad beauty may not be simply attracting male attention by her display of skin — she may also be giving the signal 'my hormones are tanked up and ready for action'!

All this gives us a rather new slant on the phenomenon of the holiday romance. After a week in the sun we feel more relaxed and therefore less inhibited, our sex hormones have been given a boost, and our whole bodies are tuned for reproduction. What's more, the opposite sex instinctively know it.

Family planning by sunlight

Remarkably, it seems that from birth onwards our sexual development and functioning is subject to regulation by sunlight. In previous chapters we discussed melatonin — the hormone produced by the pineal — which is suppressed by sunlight of sufficient brightness, and which controls the production of hormones by the pituitary gland. One of the substances regulated in this way is LH, luteinising hormone.[5] This is the hormone that causes ovulation and triggers off the second, premenstrual phase of the menstrual cycle. It also appears to influence the development of sexual maturity.

A role for the pineal gland in sexual development was first proposed in 1909 by Otto Marburg.[6] He suggested that the gland produced a chemical that inhibited sexual function, but that with age the production of this chemical would decline as the gland calcified. Since then, melatonin has been shown to suppress sexual function in some laboratory animals. In humans, the LH level is inversely proportional to the level of melatonin. As puberty progresses and body size increases, the level of melatonin decreases to its adult norm, and the level of LH rises.[7] This decline in melatonin cannot be due to calcification of the gland, which normally only happens in middle age or beyond. What does seem to happen is that the pineal produces melatonin at a steady rate over the years of growth, and the increase in body mass causes the melatonin to be progressively diluted and its effect to be reduced.[8]

Nearly all mammals have seasonal variations in their sexual habits, and seasonal cycles of fertility. However, these vary widely from species to species. So do their responses to enviromental light and to melatonin. Put as simply as it can be, mammals can be divided four ways. They are either active during the day (diurnal) or during the night (nocturnal). They are also either monoestrous, which means that they come into season only once a year, or polyoestrous, having regular ovulatory cycles throughout the year, as do humans.

Staying alive

There are obvious survival advantages to timing reproduction carefully. The most important is that if offspring can be born at a time when food is abundant they are more likely to survive – and less likely to threaten the parent animals by restricting their ability to gather food. Viewed in this light, the seasonal variation in mating, and the way this is mediated by changes in day length and therefore in total melatonin production, start to make sense.

Many small animals such as rabbits and hamsters have very short gestation (pregnancy) periods, from two weeks to two months. They mate in the spring and give birth in spring or summer. Reducing the day length, as occurs in autumn, inhibits them from breeding and so prevents them from having babies in winter. On the other hand, sheep and deer have gestation periods of six to eight months, and tend to mate in autumn and give birth in the spring. Therefore a reduction in day length causes them to come into season.[9]

In humans, the peak time for conception is late spring to early summer, leading to birth at the beginning of spring. This is not a very powerful variation, the peak rate of conception being only about ten per cent higher than the annual average.[10] It has also decreased in amplitude throughout this century. But it remains consistent for any given country. In Mediterranean Europe the peak is in April; in France, Germany, Belgium and the Netherlands it is May or June, and in Scandinavia July.

Both luteinising hormone and follicle-stimulating hormone (FSH) – the former definitely suppressed by melatonin, and the latter possibly so – show similar patterns of variation, with a spring and autumn peak in temperate climates.[11] LH also peaks at the time of ovulation, and melatonin shows a drop at the same time, which is clearly not due to sunlight levels, however, but probably to suppression of melatonin production by oestrogen.

Among most species studied, major disruptions of the day/ night cycle can interfere with the menstrual or oestrous cycle. In rats, which are nocturnal, continous illumination throughout the twenty four hours suppresses the release of LH and thereby ovulation. In humans, who are diurnal, we would expect light deficiency to do the same. There are no scientific studies yet to show that this is so, but I am not the only doctor to have seen female patients in whom light deficiency appears to disrupt and even completely stop the menstrual cycle, and in whom regular sunlight exposure produces an improvement.

Melatonin appears also to be a major factor in seasonal affective disorder, a recently recognised form of depression, which comes on particularly during the winter months. These patients are very different from the large majority of sufferers from depression, and one of the ways in which they are different is that they tend to have a different seasonal pattern of reproduction, with a peak for starting pregnancy in late summer.[12] This is scarcely surprising – presumably that is the only time they feel fit enough to get pregnant!

In winter, as in shift workers, cholesterol levels are higher. Vitamin D levels are lower, and so are steroid hormone levels. In the spring, however, the sun reappears, and we celebrate the fertility rite of Easter, with chickens and bunnies as its primal symbols, distinct from the more recent Christian ones. Everybody feels and looks better, and therefore more attractive, the conception rate hits an all-time high, the buds come out, and nature's great fertility show is on the road again. If we dare to show our faces out of doors we can join in the fun.

CHAPTER 15

Sparkling intellect – light and the brain

There are so many reasons why sunlight makes us feel better and improves our mental state that it is hard to list them all. Our brain is the most complex arrangement of cells in our body (or anywhere else on earth), and so there are, by definition, more things that can go wrong in it than in our other organs. It is energy intensive, requiring a steady supply of glucose from the blood to fuel all its operations and interactions. Minor alterations in the supply of oxygen, the flow of blood and the availability of various nutrients can all make a striking difference in brain function, which manifests itself to the sufferer as a change in the way he feels and to the observer as a change in behaviour.

Being so sensitive to biochemical changes, the brain is in many cases the best indicator there is of things going wrong. In deficiencies of the B vitamins, for example, it is most often in the brain and the central nervous system that symptoms first show. Complaints such as anxiety, fatigue, irritability, even pins and needles in the hands, are often the first signs of such a deficiency.

Because the light in which we live influences and regulates our biochemistry and our complete functioning in not just one or two, but a whole range of ways, the brain is also particularly sensitive to variations in our light intake – to light deficiency. Take a look at some examples of this.

Le Tetanie Latent

Hyperventilation is a disorder that is now recognised to be surprisingly common – and by no means only in hysterical and neurotic people. It is made more likely by some physical disorders such as allergies; victims may even wake up with the symptoms, and then have to bring it under control themselves.[1] What happens in hyperventilation is that the body reduces the oxygen supply to the brain. This is an unfortunate reflex, a minor design fault if you will, which we all have to learn how to control or cope with, but some people have much more trouble with it than others.

The supply of blood to the brain, through the carotid arteries, is regulated according to the amount of carbon dioxide in the blood coming away from the brain. The more carbon dioxide the brain produces, the more work the body deduces the brain to be performing, and so the more blood, with its cargo of oxygen, it allows in to fuel it. The carbon dioxide leaves our bodies through the lungs, but if we breathe too rapidly, we can cause an excessive loss of carbon dioxide. This leads to a signal for the body to reduce the blood flow to the brain, and consequent symptoms from lack of oxygen.

This is a simplified version of what happens, but a good working model nevertheless. Many a sufferer has tried in vain to find logical psychological explanations for the symptoms, the strange feelings, the frightening ideas that occur in hyperventilation. There are none; it is a physical phenomenon.

Hyperventilation is made significantly more likely by deficiencies of minerals, especially of magnesium. In fact, some French and other European workers regard the link as being so solid that they treat hyperventilation as a diagnostic sign of magnesium deficiency.[2] As we have seen earlier, magnesium deficiency is a very common deficiency in our society – perhaps *the* commonest. This is largely due to diet; the best source of magnesium is green vegetables, which some of us never eat from one year's end to the next! But even if we eat the things, we still need to absorb the nutrients in them, and magnesium absorption, like that of calcium, is dependent on vitamin D. We all require sunlight – and vitamin D derived from sunlight – in order to absorb and retain magnesium effectively,[3] and thereby to keep our breathing and our brains running smoothly, our nerves less jagged.

It is easy to assume that calcium is only important for bones and to forget that it is present in every cell in our body, and is a necessary part of each cell's functioning. In nerve cells, calcium has a crucial role in stimulating them to discharge, while magnesium appears to help them recover from firing. A proper balance of the two minerals is necessary for all cell function, but especially for the nervous system. A deficiency of calcium can lead to a variety of mental and neurological disorders, including depression and anxiety, insomnia, general tenseness, jumpiness and twitchiness. The symptoms of magnesium deficiency are very similar, with the addition of learning impairment, general confusion and worsening of epilepsy.[4] Both of these minerals are absorbed and conserved in the body under the regulation of vitamin D. This is best obtained from sunlight.

A bellyful of sleep

A second example is that of tryptophan metabolism. Tryptophan is the precursor of serotonin (5HT) and melatonin. Not surprisingly it has a sedative effect on humans and other animals. For instance, there is a relatively large amount of tryptophan in red meat. When large predators such as lions kill and eat their prey, they take in a hearty dose of tryptophan. This makes them drowsy and relaxed for hours or even days, during which time they doze on branches waiting to be photographed by tourists. As the tryptophan effect wears off they start to wake up, and eventually hunt for more food.

As well as regulating the sleep/wake cycle, melatonin also influences the release of endorphins in the brain. These are the naturally occuring morphine-like substances which have a controlling influence on our alertness, our appetites, and indeed our goal-oriented behaviour in general. Melatonin, derived from tryptophan, triggers the release of the sedative beta-endorphin. So at the same time as the basking lion is sent to sleep, it also loses its appetite. And which of us has not felt sleepy after a large meal?

But tryptophan is much more effective as a sedative in humans if it is given in the evening, near to bedtime. The important difference at this time, the spring in the biological clock, is production of melatonin from tryptophan, in the dark. Yet another example of light and dark interacting with the other nutrients from food to make our bodies function smoothly.

Sunlight rejuvenation

One disorder that is guaranteed to interfere with the supply of nutrients to the brain is cerebral arteriosclerosis – hardening of the arteries of the brain. In severe cases this may lead to a complete blockage of the blood supply to certain areas, with consequences such as convulsions and strokes, but more often it leads to a slow general deterioration in mental functioning and in behaviour. In Russia, the value of sunlight in treating such disorders is appreciated. A study published in 1966 on 150 patients reported that the mental functioning of cerebral arteriosclerosis sufferers was improved greatly by regular sunlight baths.[5]

The long-stay geriatric wards of many of our hospitals are full of tragic cases of people whose brains have deteriorated due to arteriosclerosis, but whose bodies carry on functioning as if all were well. They represent a considerable burden on the tax-payer, but even more they are a constant source of grief and despair to their relatives. How easy it would be to expose them all to full-spectrum light, with the necessary, nutritional, full visible and ultraviolet light components. Installing such lighting would help them all day and every day, for a cost that is quite trivial in terms of the National Health Service budget. Of course, if hospitals reverted to a slightly old-fashioned design, the patients would be able to go outside when it was sunny – but no doubt there are administrative reasons why this would be inconvenient.

Hip-hop kids

At the other extreme of the age scale, the effect of lighting on hyperactivity was first noted by Dr Ott. This is an increasing problem in schools — and homes — these days, and it has been observed to be worse under artificial lights. Since sunlight has a soothing and relaxing effect on everybody, young or old, it made sense to see whether full-spectrum lights made a difference to hyperactive children. A study was set up by a lighting company in America, and it came up with some startling results.

In a school environment which was almost entirely lit by fluorescent tubes, hyperactivity was a constant and substantial problem. But when the ordinary tubes were replaced with full-spectrum ones, things improved dramatically. These results were recorded by a hidden video camera, and studying the video brings the point home powerfully. Children who before could hardly stay on their seats started to sit down and pay attention. The rate of punishment for misbehaviour went down and the work output and learning capacity of the children went up. It was noticeable that the children who were worst to start with improved the most.[6]

As well as hospitals, it seems, we should be installing full-spectrum lights in schools. Because the pupils would feel better and be healthier physically, they would also learn better and get into less trouble.

Solar detoxification

Another Russian study looked at the body's ability to withstand poisons and eliminate them from the system. It concluded that 'tolerance of the organism to chemical substances depends, to a great extent, on its subjection to ultraviolet radiation; it drops in ultraviolet deficit and increases in exposure to suberythemic doses'. In other words, we do not need to get sunburned or even suntanned in order to experience physiological benefits from ultraviolet light.[7]

The Russians, of course, have more opportunity than us to

study ultraviolet deficit, or 'light hunger' as they have called it. They also have more reason to find treatments for it, but not that much more reason than us, since the effects of being further north are now easily outstripped by the effect of living indoors. We might as well all be in polar regions, for the amount of sunlight that we get in an ordinary day. If we adjusted our light intake upwards, this study clearly states, we would be more able to withstand the damaging effects of environmental pollution, and the pollution of our food and drink.

It has been shown that an excessive body burden of toxic minerals such as lead or cadmium can lead to high blood pressure, impairment of the functioning of the heart, and to general malaise and ill health. But the most important links by far are with hyperactivity, with behavioural and learning difficulties in children, and even with dyslexia.[8] These are growing problems, one might say. Organic molecules such as pesticides are probably even more of a problem, as it is hard to avoid them if we want to eat at all. Since a lettuce may well have been sprayed fourteen times with a range of chemicals by the time it arrives in our salad bowl, it is safe to say that we all carry a burden of pesticides and other chemicals dissolved in our fatty tissues. These chemicals operate as neurotoxins. They kill pests by poisoning their nervous system and paralysing them. But if the pest has a nervous system, then it is similar to humans, at least in that respect, and there is no reason why we should be immune to the neurotoxic effects.

Pesticide residues have been incriminated in cases of psychological illness, even more so of chronic fatigue, depression and general malaise, and in extreme cases of triggering allergies. In some way that we do not yet appreciate, they damage the immune system, and can lead to the development of severe and fulminating allergy problems.[9] If our ability to tolerate and resist the damaging effects of these chemicals is proportional to our exposure to ultraviolet light, then we have a major treatment ready and waiting for what is clearly an increasing health problem.

Patients who have been found to have high body burdens of

toxic chemicals could benefit from sunlight or full-spectrum light by an increase in their excretion of these toxins. But prevention is always better than cure, and it is more important still to ensure our children get enough sunlight to keep their load of toxins down and prevent such illnesses from developing.

Strategic secretions

Exposure to sunlight also stimulates the output of our thyroid glands. Since the thyroid hormones regulate the metabolic rate, this can have a dramatic, although subtle and sometimes easy to miss, effect on the way we feel. Patients with even mild hypothyroidism (low thyroid hormone output) often feel chronically fatigued, rundown, unable to concentrate, generally unwell, and in need of excessive sleep. They also tend to put on weight, which can depress them still further.[10] Sunlight, through the pineal-pituitary axis, can increase the output of the thyroid gland and remedy these problems.

By the same mechanism, it can stimulate the output of the adrenal gland. Adrenal products fall into two categories; the long-acting corticosteroid hormones, which have effects on the whole of our metabolism; and the short-acting chemicals, such as adrenaline, which are released into the bloodstream and have immediate effects on blood pressure, heart rate, general arousal level, and ability to cope with stress and emergencies. Patients with poor adrenal output tend to suffer from a drop in blood pressure on standing up. This is the simplest model imaginable of a failure to adapt to a change in circumstances. When we stand up, the height of the column of blood in which we have to maintain pressure, and circulation, may double or treble. A small release of adrenaline is required in order to adjust the pressure. Sufferers from hypoadrenalism cannot provide this.

They also suffer from chronically low energy levels, susceptibility to infection, poor temperature regulation and chronic backache, and generally feel lousy.[11] In Chapter 12, I mentioned the experiments on adrenal steroid output under different lighting conducted by Hollwich. He found that in daylight healthy subjects kept a normal, healthy output of ACTH from the pituitary and cortisol from the adrenal. But under artificial light of the ordinary type, output climbed within two weeks to a stress level.

It is a well understood fact that if the production of an endocrine gland is pushed up to abnormally high levels for any length of time, the gland may become exhausted and depleted of nutrients. A second, exhaustion phase, with lowered output and inability to respond to minor increases in demand, can ensue. Hypoadrenalism is an example of this. Increased exposure to sunlight can help to stabilise the output of the adrenal to normal levels. It should be a component of any treatment programme for adrenal insufficiency, and of everybody's plan for staying healthy.

A question of wavelengths

Another problem with living indoors is that of visual fatigue. Anybody working indoors, particularly at office work, suffers eye strain at times. One of the reasons for this is that the light reaching the eye is refracted differently according to its wavelength. There is a difference in the refraction between red and violet of about 2 dioptres, which is a reasonably powered pair of spectacles. This means that a correct focus for one colour of light may be several centimetres out for another colour.

As a result our eyes may be constantly trying to adapt and adjust their focus, but never succeed. The more distorted the light source the more serious this problem can be. This was brought out in an American study which looked at the 'spectral effectiveness factor'. This is a more or less incomprehensible mathmatical product based on the number of mistakes that are made in visual tasks under that light. They found a difference of just over 22 per cent between a good light and a bad light. The good light, it seems, is always the light with the broadest spectrum, and therefore the nearest replication of natural daylight.[12]

Another study looked at fatigue and visual acuity under two

different lights – regular fluorescent and full-spectrum. They found that under ordinary lights people reported feeling fatigued after the set period of four hours, but under FSL they did not. When they measured visual acuity – the sharpness of vision – it actually improved under FSL, but worsened under normal lighting.[13]

The implications of this for anybody who employs personnel to do paperwork or look at computer screens for long periods of time, for example, or for anybody engaged in study, are quite staggering, The implications for all of us who have to live under such lighting are equally disturbing. Very few of us are able to arrange our lives so that we can work under sunlight, so attempts to improve the quality of indoor lighting are clearly called for.

Blue February

In this chapter I have deliberately avoided so far the subject of SAD, Seasonal Affective Disorder. In the form that it is now recognised by doctors, this is relatively unusual. It certainly responds to bright light of a composition near to daylight. It certainly also represents an abnormally high requirement for light as a nutrient. But I would not like you to think that there is a tiny number of people with SAD who need large quantities of light to stay cheerful, and the rest of us are doing fine. Far from it.

The fact that individual needs for particular vitamins vary widely from person to person was clearly and conclusively shown some years ago – first by Roger Williams, who is in many ways the founder of nutritional medicine. Because of the immense variety in our genes and therefore our biochemistry, one human may require several times more vitamin B6, for example, than the next in order to stay well. Another may need more vitamin B12, or more zinc, and so on. The same applies to light. For every sufferer from SAD there will be many who experience less clear-cut, but still damaging, mental symptoms in low-light conditions. And there will be others who cannot produce enough vitamin D, and so develop calcium or magnesium deficiencies. Negro and Asian people, for instance, are especially likely to have this problem.

But most importantly, we *all* live in poor light environments these days, unless we work outside regularly. We could all benefit from more light in our diet. As George Somerville, MD said 50 years ago;

The beneficial light of the sun, winter and summer, induces an intimate emotional satisfaction – a pleasing expansion of the whole being which creates a healthy outlook on life.

CHAPTER 16

Colour me healthy

Another book could be written – and several have – on the component colours of daylight and their different effects on us. A considerable science has grown up based on colour psychology and there is no question that some very powerful changes can be wrought in our state of mind, and our state of body, by skilful use of colours.

Until very recently in man's development, the theory states, all our colours were derived from nature. The green of the leaves, the blue of the sky, the colours of flowers and animals, were all that our eyes saw. It was not until the industrial revolution, and the mass production of fabrics, that synthetic dyes became widely available – although a limited amount of dyeing has gone on in some societies for hundreds of years. Because of the expense, the labour involved and the relative rarity of the raw materials for dyes, coloured fabrics tended to be the prerogative of the ruling caste. More often than not, interestingly, the only dye available appears to have been purple. This association of purple with royalty has entered our own culture.

Nowadays, colours are widely available to all of us in clothing, paints and wallpapers, packaging and many other aspects of the environment. We tend to choose colours for aesthetic reasons or because they are fashionable, and easily forget that they can have a profound psychological impact. Colour psychologists, however, who work in the advertising industry more than anywhere else, have not forgotten this. They use selection of colour as a way of fine-tuning our response to a variety of products and ideas.

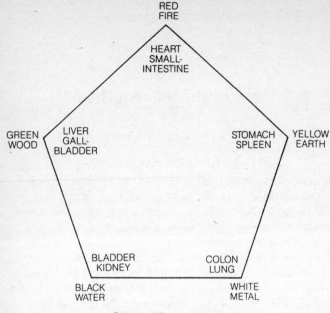

Chinese 5 Element System

A patchwork of light

An interesting sideline on this is provided by the founders of the succesful American clothing company Esprit, which recently opened its first stores in Britain. Their high-fashion 'leisurewear' is notable for its use of strong, bright colours. Yet the couple who started Esprit are among the leading collectors of antique American quilts. The walls of their open-plan offices in San Francisco are decorated with these beautiful, subtly patterned quilts, many of them made by the Amish sect, who completely reject the use of synthetic dyes in their fabrics. The dark, muted colours they use have a surprisingly soothing effect. Yet Esprit say that they derive inspiration from them for their ultra-modern designs.

The ups and downs

The most basic differentiation of colour derives from the day/ night cycle, which controls our pineal melatonin output, and all our other rhythms as well. Put simply, there is a time (daytime) for activity, for expending energy, for the pursuit of food and other interests. There is also a time (night-time) for rest, retreat into our cave or hut, and repair of our bodies and minds.[1] There is a cycle within our metabolism that tunes to this day/night cycle, whereby in the morning our bodies are catabolising, which is to say using up and breaking down the component molecules of our cells to fuel our energy expenditure. At the same time, waste components are filtered out and excreted. In the evening and night, on the other hand, we enter an anabolic phase, during which we repair and build up our cell structures, providing healing and recovery.[2]

The theory of colour psychology states quite simply that we will respond positively to a colour that corresponds with our physical or psychological need. If we are in need of rest, calm, relaxation and healing, we will choose a dark, night time colour. If on the other hand we seek energetic pursuits, ambitious stri- vings and the satisfaction of our appetites, we will go for a brighter daytime colour.

In the Luscher colour test, for instance, states of mind and emotional conflicts, even physical illnesses, can be detected from the way people respond to colours. A series of coloured cards are presented to the person to be tested, who chooses the one most preferred, and then the one most preferred of those remaining, and so on to the last. The sequence of choices provides a surprisingly detailed and logical insight into the person's psychology.[3] In the short version of this test, eight colours are used, so there are 40,320 possible different sequences.

There is a scale of colours from the most outgoing, stimulus- seeking colour, yellow, to the most retiring, calm-seeking, blue. There is even a list of diseases which are commonly associated with notable choice of each colour. The test can therefore be used to identify psychological stresses and problems, and their physical consequences too. As a psychological tool, it has been used in medicine and industry by a number of people with notable success.

Seeing red

In recent years researchers, particularly in the social sciences, have turned the problem round and looked at it from the opposite direction. They have reasoned that if colours can be used to detect states of mind, perhaps they can also be used to influence them. A West German study using college students found that the use of yellow, orange or red colours in the classroom produced an increase in IQ and academic achievement. The use of brown or black suppressed these abilities.[4]

John Ott uncovered an interesting angle on this when he gave a lecture in Florida nearly twenty years ago. Afterwards he was approached by the manager of a local radio station, who told him of their remarkable experience with office lighting. In an attempt to brighten up the office, the regular fluorescent tubes in the studios and control rooms had been replaced with deep pink ones. After a few weeks, everybody there started to show signs of strain. People were more irritable, argued about everything and objected to every management decision even without grounds. The announcers started making mistakes and performing badly on air.

It wasn't until several more weeks had passed, and two of the staff had resigned for no clear reason, that the penny dropped. When one staff member complained about the pink lights specifically, management immediately had them replaced with white ones. Two weeks later everyone had returned to normal, tempers had settled down, and the resignations had been withdrawn. The announcers were even performing well on air again.[5]

Dr Ott immediately saw the connection with another experiment in which he had been involved, at a mink farm in Illinois. Different cages of mink were kept behind different colours of glass or plastic. Those with blue tints to their cages became strikingly docile and friendly – and anyone who has ever handled a mink will attest to how unfriendly they are. But those in the pink-shaded cages became even more aggressive and dangerous. There were effects on reproduction too, with those in the blue area becoming more fertile, and those in pink areas having less litters than normal. The natural deduction from this is that mink respond to blue environments better because they orginally come from well up in the north of Canada, where the nights are long and dark, and they hunt by night. Humans, of course, originate from East Africa.

Psycho-colour

The use of environmental colour has now been considerably refined, most noticeably by Professor Harry Wohlfarth at the University of Edmonton, in Alberta. He has conducted a number of studies in schools and work places.[6] He finds that the colour scheme outlined in theoretical colour psychology – with yellow and red as the most stimulating colours, and blue and black as the most calming – holds fast. He has used blue walls to calm down hyperactive children, to lower blood pressure and reduce stress in general.[7] Yellow, on the other hand, has been found to increase alertness and learning ability. There is in fact a clear-cut scale of effects, from most to least stimulating.

As well as influencing the psychological state, this colour system has been shown to affect blood pressure, pulse and respiration rates. Remarkably, it appears to be just as effective in people who are colour-blind. The same applies to the Luscher colour test. This is taken to be evidence that the mechanism operating here is physiological rather than psychological. On the other hand these colour psychodynamic effects, as they have come to be termed, do require the accurate colour rendering provided by sunlight or full-spectrum lighting for their full impact.

Pretty in Pink

One of the most powerful demonstrations of the use of colour was conducted in a US Marine correctional centre in Seattle, Washington State. The military police at this camp had a lock-up for arrested men while the paperwork for charging them was prepared. They were likely to be in there for something less than an hour. This room had always been the site of frequent disturbances. Men detained in it regularly became abusive and even violent. Many of them, of course, were roaring drunk when put in there.

The colour psychodynamic measure proposed for this room was extremely simple. It was to be painted pink. The colour in question was a precise hue, reputedly the colour which would be perceived by a baby in the womb. After the colour change, disturbances and outbursts in this cell decreased almost to nil. The effect was dramatic and unarguable.[8]

Since then, the use of Baker-Miller pink, as it has come to be known, after two of the major participants in the original study, has become relatively common throughout the USA and Canada as a means of calming aggressive or agitated inmates in institutions and prisons. It is even used by a number of sheriffs' offices in the lock-ups to which Saturday night drunks are committed. Everybody employing the technique reports excellent results.

There is one drawback: an overdose can be dangerous. When men were left in the pink room for about two hours, some of

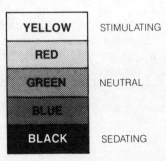

them became very disturbed and made self-destructive attempts. Clearly the sedating effect is capable of building up to the extent of severe depression. If anything, this is further proof of the potency of colour in changing the way that we think and feel.

Colour psychodynamics will grow in importance, and we will all eventually find ourselves exposed sometimes to its colour schemes. You may feel that this is manipulation of your mind, but for myself I would rather work in an office which has been designed and colour-schemed with some of my physiological and psychological needs in mind, than in one that is merely the product of an architect's whim.

The new information on light and colour, on their essentiality, their health benefits, their specific physiological effects, provides us all with an opportunity to rework our environment. Each of us can take this chance or leave it. We can modify our lifestyle, change our indoor lighting and put pressure on our employers to do the same, or we can continue to fungate in the dark. Bearing in mind a magical figure that has recurred several times throughout this text, *it is likely that by using sunlight and full-spectrum light together, plus some commonsense adjustments to our lifestyles and sensible nutrition, we can make our lives 2.5 times more liveable.*

What to do

If we believe that sunlight is good for us, then we need to work out what to do about it. In this section I will try to give you some guidelines.

Put simply, there are two things you can do to correct a light deficiency. You can get more sunlight, or you can use an artificial source. My advice is to do both. After all, there are only a limited number of days when there's any sunlight to speak of in this country. And we know that much of the population is chronically short of UV, especially in winter. It makes sense to take measures to keep up your exposure during the winter, and many of us find it impossible to escape from work into the sun in summer.

Out of the frying pan

Let's look first at ways of using the sun. The first and most vital rule has to be:

DON'T GET BURNED

Sunburn may not be the root of all evil, but it definitely does age the skin and release free oxidising radicals into the body which can make us ill in various ways. If we are exposed repeatedly over many years, it can lead to skin cancer. So, it makes all the sense in the world to avoid it.

Sunplanning

The way to avoid sunburn is quite simple: start gradually, be methodical. Our skin has its own designed-in protection against burning, after all, in the form of a suntan. It just needs time to build up this protection; during this time your skin can only handle small doses of ultraviolet.

The other factor that you have to bear in mind is your skin type. People of Celtic extraction very commonly have skin which hardly tans at all and is very prone to burning. They consequently need much less time in the sun. But with patient, cautious exposure they *can* build up a tolerance to sunlight, and this is worth doing as it makes it possible to get more of the beneficial effects of the sun.

The first step is to calculate your personal starting dose. By using Table 1 below you can work out how long *in bright direct sunlight* in July in England you are likely to need to just start burning – your minimal erythema dose, or MED. From Russian research, we know that the best starting dose is about half of the MED. So when you have worked out your personal MED, halve it, and that is your starting time for July.

Table 1

TYPE	mJ/cm^2 MED	TIME
I	25-30	20 Minutes
II	25-35	30 Minutes
III	30-50	40 Minutes
IV	45-60	50 Minutes
V	60-80	70 Minutes
VI	80-200	140 Minutes

Next you have to allow for the fact that the amount of sun around goes down dramatically as we move into autumn or spring. From November to February there probably isn't enough sun in Britain to tan or burn anybody. Table 2 shows how the time needed to get an MED goes up at these times of the year. It is based on somebody with a Type Two skin, not recently tanned, who would normally need about half an hour in July to start to burn.

Table 2

Month	Time Needed	Time Available	
January	Unlimited	None	
February	Unlimited	None	
March	6 Hours	11am-1pm	
April	2½ Hours	10am-2pm	
May	1 Hour	9am-3pm	
June	45 Minutes		Tanning
July	30 Minutes	8am-4pm	Possible
August	40 Minutes		
September	1¼ Hours	10am-2pm	
October	3½ Hours	11am-1pm	
November	Unlimited	None	
December	Unlimited	None	

You can also allow yourself longer if the sky is overcast or cloudy, or you are sitting in the shade. Table 3 shows how the UV in sunlight is reduced, but not completely cut out, by cloud and shade. So it may still be possible to benefit, even on a cloudy day.

If you are going abroad, say to the Mediterranean, you can easily adjust your timing. In fact, the intensity of sunlight in summer is not that much greater than in Britain – it's just that there are more hours of cloudless sky in an average day in Crete or the Costa Brava than in Cambridge. Also the level of light intensity stays up at summer levels for longer – from about March to September rather than June to August. So use the same calculation as for July in Britain. For Africa or other tropical areas, reduce your time by one third.

Table 3

	UV Reduced To	Increase Exposure By
DIRECT	100%	0%
SHADE	60%	60%
OVERCAST	80%	25%
CLOUDY	50%	50%

Setting out

Before you start sunbathing, work out how long you need for your starting dose. You can then increase this by about a minute per day for bright sun, or two for indirect sun. Always halt the increase for a week if you experience any burning, and stay out of the sun until the burn has settled down.

The only essential piece of equipment is a clock or watch, so that you can time your exposure. No creams or sunscreens are needed, in fact they are a positively bad idea. They block out the UV, which rather defeats the whole purpose of being there at all, and they do carry a risk of causing skin rashes.

There is no reason why you have to be lying down to take in sunlight. Indeed, there is always the possibility that, if lying down, you will fall asleep and overdo it. Gardening, or playing a ball game, or just pottering about, are all eminently suitable.

The only danger is that if you become absorbed in a tough set of tennis, or in rescuing your hydrangeas, you may still leave one part of your skin exposed to the sun for so long that you burn.

The other point about lying down is that we generally find it more natural to remove items of clothing when lying than when walking about. Since the effects of UV on the body as a whole increase with the amount of skin bared, this is generally a good idea. The degree of benefit varies according to a simple sum:

EFFECT

=

INTENSITY OF LIGHT REACHING SKIN

times

LENGTH OF TIME EXPOSED

times

SKIN AREA EXPOSED

So it must be beneficial to remove as many clothes as possible – without risking hypothermia or arrest. If, as is so often the case, the weather does not allow undressing, you can still get some benefit, particularly that from sunlight entering the eye, simply by being outside. So it may well pay you to get a dog, who will require to be walked even at times when you would rather not, or a garden which will reproach you just as much if you fail to get out there and tend it.

The last point that you must remember is that glasses, including sunglasses and contact lenses, all filter out the UV. John Ott discovered the therapeutic use of breaking your glasses for himself, and has since applied it to many other people. Until it becomes possible to obtain ultraviolet-transmitting spectacles in this country, I have to advise you to step outside without any lenses if at all possible. This particularly applies to sunglasses, of course.

On the other hand, hats appear to be having something of a

revival, it is pleasant to observe. Hats have the definite edge over sunglasses in that they cut out most of the glare without blocking the UV. They also offer great scope for imaginative statements about oneself.

Indoor sunlight

Whether you can or cannot get out in the sun, it is still going to be worth your while investing in some full-spectrum lighting. This can be installed anywhere that you are going to spend time, and has the advantage of providing the benefits of sunlight without the risk of burning, and without the necessity of stepping out of doors to experience it. With recent advances in design, it is also possible to obtain lights that eliminate most of the other potential risks of ordinary fluorescent lights, such as radiation leakage from the electric poles.

There are two different approaches: one for sufferers from seasonal affective disorder, and one for the rest of us. SAD sufferers need a minimum intensity of 2500 lux, which is *very* bright light by indoor standards, to suppress melatonin production in the pineal gland. This is far less important for people without the problem.

The brightness goes down sharply the further away you are from a light source, according to what physicists call the Inverse Square Law. That is to say, if you halve your distance from the source, you quadruple the intensity. For example, doubling the distance from two feet to four feet will reduce the intensity to one quarter of what it was. Trebling distance will reduce it ninefold. So the rule for SAD sufferers is to install the light in such a way that you can get very close to it – with your eyes about a foot away.

Use the light as an ordinary source of illumination throughout the day, but also go within a foot of it for regular spells. You do not need to look straight into the light, as light will get in through the iris and the pupil at an oblique angle. With a bit of trial and error you will be able to gauge your own needs in terms of time spent up close to the light. It will probably be about twenty minutes, but some people find that five minutes is sufficient, while others seem to need an hour.

Try to time these 'mega-doses' so that they bracket your day – one in the early morning and one in the evening. It is possible that you will need more doses during the day, but you will find this out for yourself. Even if you need several doses, make sure that you keep up the morning and evening treatments.

Preventive lighting

For those of us without winter depression, life is a lot simpler. We don't need to cuddle up to a lamp, we can just install it and live and work under it. There will still be an advantage from having as much light intensity as possible, because our eyes adapt over a great range, and we fail to realise that normal indoor lighting is really very dim indeed. If we raised that level of brightness using regular lights, then we would only compound the problems that these lights cause. But with full-spectrum lighting, an increase in intensity should bring an increase in benefits. So it pays to put in as many lights as you can reasonably manage.

Whatever your problem, you may well benefit also from exposing your whole body sometimes, not just your head – from lightbathing in fact. If your are able to set up a light in such a way that you can lie or stand unclothed within a couple of feet of it occasionally, then you can hope to unclog your system, stimulate the circulation, tone up your muscles, detoxify yourself and boost your production of vitamin D and hormones. All the benefits of sunlight, in fact, but at a lower dosage.

Whatever your problem, and whatever approach you adopt to treating it, I can only hope that you get real benefit from sunlight, and enjoy yourself at the same time. I'll see you out there.

References

Chapter one

1 Wyke, Alexandra, 'Molecules and Market', *The Economist*, Vol. 306, no. 7484, Feb 1987.
2 Ott, John, *'My Ivory Cellar'*, Twentieth Century Press, Chicago, 1958.
3 Ott John, *Health and Light*, Pocket Books, New York, 1973.

Chapter two

1 Metzler, D. E., *Biochemistry: The Chemical Reactions of Living Cells*, Academic Press, New York, 1977.
2 Porter, G., and Archer M., 'In Vitro Photosynthesis', *Interdisciplinary Science Reviews:* 1 no. 2, Heyden & Sons, 1976.

Chapter three

1 Thorington, L., 'Spectral Irradiance and Temporal Aspects of Natural and Artificial Light', *Ann. New York Acad. Sci:* 435; 28–54, 1985.
2 IES Lighting Handbook, 1981.
3 Wurtman, R.J., and Moskowitz, M.A., 'The Pineal Organ', *The New England Journal of Medicine* 296; 23; 1329–1333, 1977.
4 Okudaira, N., Kripke, D.F., and Webster, J.B., 'Naturalistic Studies of Human Light Exposure', *American Journal of Physiology*, 245: R613–R615, 1983.

5 Wever, R.A., *The Circadian System of Man*, Springer-Verlag, New York, 1979.

6 Wever, R.A., 'Use of Light To Treat Jet Lag: Differential Effects of Normal and Bright Artificial Light on Human Circadian Rhythms', *Ann. New York Acad. Sci:* 435; 282–304, 1985.

7 Rosenthal, N.E., et al., 'Seasonal Affective Disorder and Phototherapy' *Ann. New York Acad. Sci:* 435; 254–260, 1985.

8 Lawson. D.E.M., and Davies, M.J.W., *Vitam. Horm.* 39,1., 1980.

9 Dantsig, M., *Effect and Use of Ultraviolet Radiation (Ultrafioletovoye Izulcheniya),* Meditsina Publishing House, Moscow, 1966.

Chapter four

1 Wever, R.A., 'Use of Light to Treat Jet Lag: Differential Effects of Normal and Bright Artificial Light on Human Circadian Rhythms', *Ann. New York Acad. Sci:* 435; 282–304, 1985.

2 Velikovsky, I., *Worlds in Collision*, Gollancz, London, 1950.

3 Leiberman, H.R., et al., 'Possible Behavioural Consequences of Light Induced Changes in Melanoma Availablity', *Ann. New York Acad. Sci:* 435; 242–252, 1985.

4 Erlich, S., et al. 'The Pineal Gland; Anatomy, Physiology and Clinical Significance', *Journal of Neurosurgery*: 1985; 321–341, 1985.

5 Williams, R., 'Pineal Gland', *Textbook of Endocrinology* 6th ed., W.B. Saunders Co., Philadelphia, 1981.

6 Pfeiffer, C., 'Zinc and Other Micronutrients'.

7 Wever, R.A., *The Circadian System of Man*, Springer-Verlag, New York, 1979.

8 Cremer-Bartels, G., et al., 'Magnetic Field of the Earth as

Additional Zeitgeber for Endogenous Rhythms?',
Naturwissenschaften: 71; 567–574, 1986.

9 Wurtman, R.J., 'The Effects of Light on Man and Other Mammals', *Annual Review of Physiology*: 37; 467–483, 1975.

10 Wurtman, R.J., and Moskowitz, M.A., 'The Pineal Organ', *New England Journal of Medicine*: 296; 1329–1333, 1977.

11 Brainard, G.C., et al., 'Effect of Light Wavelength on the Suppression of Nocturnal Plasma Melatonin in Normal Volunteers', *Ann. New York Acad. Sci:* 435; 376–378, 1985.

12 Dietzel, M., et al., 'Effects of Bright Light and Practical Sleep Deprivation', *7th European Sleep Congress Abstracts:* 335, Munich, 1984.

13 Rosenthal, N.E, et al., 'Seasonal Affective Disorder and Phototherapy', *Ann. New York Acad. Sci:* 435; 260–267, 1985.

14 Aschoff, J., 'Annual Rhythms in Man', in Aschoff, J. (ed.), *Handbook of Behavioural Neurobiology,* Plenum Press, New York, 1981.

15 Myerson, A., and Neustadt, R., 'Influence of Ultraviolet Irradiation upon Excretion of Sex Hormones In the Male', *Endocrinology:* 25; 7, 1939.

16 Shaw, K.A, 'The Pineal Gland: A Review'.

17 Darnall, L., 'The Pineal Gland and Ageing', *Complementary Medicine:* 2 no. 2; 4751, 1986.

Chapter five

1 Mellanby, E., 'The Part Played by an "Accessory Factor" in the Production of Experimental Rickets' *Journal of Physiology*, 52: 1114, 1918.

2 Holick, M.F., et al., 'Photochemistry and Photobiology of Vitamin D', *Photomedicine*, Regan and Parrish (eds): 195–218, Plenum Press, New York, 1982.

3 Owen, I., 'Geographical Distribution of Rickets, Acute and

Subacute Rheumatism, Chorea, Cancer, and Urinary Calculus in the British Islands', *British Medical Journal*: 1; 113–116, 1889.

4 Steenbock, H., and Black, A., 'The Reduction of Growth Promoting and Calcifying Properties in a Ration by Exposure to UV Light'. *J. Biol. Chem.*: 62; 408–422, 1924.

5 Lawson D.E.M., 'Vitamin D' in Diplock, A.T. (ed.), *Fat Soluble Vitamins*, Heinemann, London, 1985.

6 Morgan, K.J., et al., 'Magnesium and Calcium Dietary Intakes of the U.S. Population', *Journal of the American College of Nutrition*,4; 195, 1985.

7 Lawson, D.E.M., in Diplock, A.T. (ed.), *Fat Soluble Vitamins,* Heinemann, London, 1985.

8 Malm, O.J., 'Calcium Requirement and Adaptation in Man', *Scand. J. Clin. Lab Invest.* 10: Suppl 36, 1958.

9 *The Nutritional Desk Reference*, Keats, New York, 1985.

10 Sharp, G.S., and Fisher, H.W., 'The Diagnosis and Treatment of Achlorhydria: Ten Year Study', *Journal of the American Geriatic Society*: 15; 786, 1967.

11 Bray, G.W., 'The Hypochlorhydria of Asthma in Childhood', *Q.J. Med.* January 1931, 1881.

12 Lutwak, L., 'The Role of Dietary Calcium/Phosphorus Ratio in Human Nutrition'. Proceedings of the Meat Industry Research Conference, 21 March, 1975.

13 Davies, S., and Stewart, A., '*Nutritional Medicine*', Pan Books, London 1987.

14 Abraham, G.E., 'The Calcium Controversy' *Journal of Applied Nutrition,*; 34,2; 69–73, 1982.

15 Gaby, A.R. and Wright, J.V., 'Nutritional Therapy in Medical Practice' Seminar, The Wright/Gaby Nutrition Institute, Baltimore, 1986.

16 Barzel, U.S., 'Acid Loading and Osteoporosis', *Journal of the American Geriatic Society*: 30; 613, 1982.

17 East, B.R., 'Mean Annual Hours of Sunshine and the Incidence of Dental Caries', *American Journal of Public Health*; 29; 777, 1939.

18 Metzler, D.E., *'Biochemistry: The Chemical Reaction of Living Cells'*, Academic Press, New York, 1977.

19 Albanese, A.A., et al., 'Effects of Calcium Supplements on Serum Cholesterol, Calcium, Phosphorus and Bone Density of "Normal, Healthy" Elderly Females', Nut. Rep. Int: 8; 119, 1973.

20 Selye, H., *Calciphylaxis*, University of Chicago Press, 1962.

21 Neer, R.M., et al., 'Environmental and Nutritional Influences on Plasma Hydroxyvitamin D Concentrations and Calcium Metabolism in Man', Norman, A.N., et al. (eds): 595–606 in *Vitamin D: Biochemical, Chemical and Clinical Aspects Related to Calcium Metabolism*, Walter de Gruyter, Berlin.

22 Lawson, D.E.M., et al., 'The Relative Contributions of Diet and Sunlight to Vitamin D State in the Elderly', *British Medical Journal*: ii; 303, 1979.

23 Doppelt, S.H., et al., 'Osteomalacia and Vitamin D Deficiency in Patients with Hip Fractures: An Unrecognised Epidemic' (abstract), American Academy of Orthopaedic Surgeons Annual Meeting.

24 Neer, R.M., 'Stimulation by Artificial Lighting of Calcium Absorption in Elderly Human Subjects', *Nature*, Vol 229, January 1971.

25 Maxwell, D., 'Subclinical and Overt Vitamin D Deficiency', Nutrition in General Practice 1, 6th BSNM Conference, London, November 1986.

26 East, B.R., 'Mean Annual Hours of Sunshine and Incidence of Dental Caries', *American Journal of Public Health*, Vol 29, July 1939.

27 Davies, D.M., 'Calcium Metabolism in Healthy Men Deprived of Sunlight', *Ann. New York Acad. Sci*: 453; 21–27, 1985.

Chapter six

1 Ott, John, *Health and Light*, Pocket Books, New York, 1973.

2 Peller, S., 'Skin Irradiation and Cancer in the U.S. Navy', *American Journal of Medical Science*: 194; 326–333, 1937.

3 Hoffman, F.L., *The Mortality of Cancer Throughout the World*, Appendix E, Prudential Press, 1915.

4 Apperly, F.L., 'The Relation of Solar Radiation to Cancer Mortality in North America', Cancer Research.

5 Garland, C., et al., 'Dietary Vitamin D and Calcium and Risk of Colorectal Cancer', *Lancet:* I; 307–309, 1985.

Chapter seven

1 Cramer, W., 'The Prevention of Cancer', *Lancet*: I; 15, 1934.

2 Fry, J., Sandler, G., and Brooks, D., *Disease Data Book*, MTP Press Ltd., Lancaster, 1986.

3 Green, A., and Siskind, V., 'Geographical Distribution of Cutaneous Melanoma in Queensland', *The Medical Journal of Australia*, April 1983.

4 Beral, V., et al., 'Malignant Melanoma and Exposure to Fluorescent Lighting at Work'. *Lancet*, 7 August 1982.

5 Pasternak, B.S., 'Malignant Melanoma and Exposure to Fluorescent Lighting at Work', *Lancet*, 26 March 1983.

6 Holman, C.D.J., and Armstrong, B.K., 'Relationship of Cutaneous Malignant Melanoma to Individual Sunlight Exposure Habits', *Journal of the National Cancer Institute*, Vol 76, No 3, March 1986.

7 Elwood, J.M., et al., 'Sun Exposure and Malignant Melanoma', *Br. J. Cancer*: 51; 543549, 1985.

8 MacKie, R.M., 'Links Between Exposure to UV Radiation and Skin Cancer', *Journal of the Royal College of Physicians*, Vol 21 No. 2, April 1987.

9 Colston, K., et al., 1, 25 – Dihydroxyvitamin D and malignant Melanoma: The Presence of Receptors and Inhibition of Cell Growth in Culture', *Endocrinology*: 108; 1083–83, 1981.

10 Pasternak, B.S., et al., 'Malignant Melanoma and Exposure

to Fluorescent Lighting at Work' (Letter) *Lancet:* 1; 704, 1983.

11 MacKie, R.M., et al., 'Malignant Melanoma in Scotland 1979–1983'. *Lancet:* 2; 859–862, 1985.

12 Hodges, N.D.M., et al., 'Evidence for Increased Genetic Damage due to the Presence of a Sunscreen Agent', *J. Pharm. Pharmacol:* 28; 53, 1976.

13 Apperley, F.L., 'The Relation of Solar Radiation to Cancer Mortality in North America', *Cancer Research.*

14 Conrad, K.K., and Hill A.B., 'Mortality from Cancer of the Skin in Relation to Mortality from Cancer of Other Sites'. *Am. J. Cancer:* 36; 8397, 1939.

15 Coyle, J.D., Hill, R.R., and Roberts, D.R. (eds), *Light, Chemical Change and Life*, Open University Press, Milton Keynes, 1982.

16 Ott, John, *Health and Light*, Pocket Books, New York, 1973.

17 Achey, P.M., et al., 'Photoreactivation of Pyrimidine Dimers in DNA, from Thyroid Cells of the Teleost Poccilia Formosa'. *Photochem Photobiol:* 29; 305–310, 1979.

18 Sutherland, B.M., 'Pyrimidine Dimer Formation and Repair in Human Skin'. *Cancer Research:* 40; 3181–3185, 1980.

19 Sutherland, B.M., 'Photoreactivation and Other Ultraviolet/Visible Light Effects on DNA in Human Skin', *Ann. N.Y. Acad. Sci:* 453; 73–79, 1985.

20 Pathak, M.A., 'Activation of the Melanocyte System by Ultraviolet Radiation and Cell Transformation', *Ann. N.Y. Acad. Sci:* 453; 328–339, 1985.

Chapter eight

1 New Gurwitsch.

2 Gurwitsch, A., 'Die Natur des Specifischen Erregurs der Zellteilung', *Roux, Archiv:* 100; 11, 1923.

3 Siebert, W.W., 'Uber die mitogenetische Strahlung des

Arbeitsmuskels and einiger anderer Gewebe', *Biochem Z*: 202; 115, 1928.

4 Wolff, L.K., and Ras, G., 'Uber die Methodik zum Nachweis der Gurwitschstrahlen', *Centr. f. Bakt I. Orig*: 128; 314, 1933.

5 Braunstein, A.E., and Heyfetz, P.A., 'Die Glycolyse und die mitogenetische Strahlung des Bluts bei experimentellen Carcinoma', *Biochem Z: 259*; 175, 1933.

6 Rahn, O., *Invisible Radiations of Organisms*, Borntraeger, Berlin, 1936.

7 Wolff, L.K., and Ras, G., 'Uber mitogenetische Strahlen: IV. Uber Sekunderstrahlung', *Centr. f. Bakt. I. Orig:* 128; 306, 1933.

8 Gesenius, H., 'Blutstrahlung and Carcinom-Diagnostik' *Radiobiologia*: 1; 33, 1932.

Chapter nine

1 Knott, E.K., 'Development of Ultraviolet Blood Irradiation', *Am. J. Surgery:* LXXVI, No 2; 165–171, 1948.

2 Miley, G., 'Ultraviolet Blood Irradiation in Acute Pyogamic Infections', *Am. J. Surgery:* LVII No 3; 493–507, 1942.

3 Schwartz, S.O., et al., 'Ultraviolet Irradiation of Blood in Man', *Journal of the American Medical Association*, 149 No 13; 1180–1184, 1952.

4 Gurwitsch, A., 'L' Analyse mitogenetique spectrale', *Exposès de Physiolgie* Vol IV; Hermann, Paris, 1934.

5 Downes A., and Blunt T.P., 'Researches on the Effect of Light upon Bacteria and Other Organisms', *Proceedings of the Royal Society of Medicine*, 26; 488, 1877.

6 Phillipson, S.M., *Germicidal Radiation and its Applications*, Thorn Lighting Company.

7 Thorington, L., 'Spectral Irradiance and Temporal Aspects of Natural and Artificial Light', *Ann. N.Y. Acad. Sci*: 453; 28–54, 1985.

8 Miley, G., 'The Knott Technique of UV blood irradiation', *New York Journal of Medicine*: 42; 38–46, 1942.

9 Ronge, H.E., 'Ultraviolet Irradiation with Artificial Illumination: A Technical, Physiological and Hygienic Study', *Acta Physiol Scand:* 15 (supp. 49); 163–171, 1948.

10 Wheeler, S.M., et al. 'Ultraviolet Light Control of Airborne Infections in a Naval Training Center', *American Journal of Public Health*: 35; 457–468, 1945.

11 Allen, R.M., Cureton, T.K., 'Effect of Ultraviolet Radiation on Physical Fitness', *Arch Phys Med:* 26; 641–644, 1945.

12 Belyager, I.I., et al, 'Combined use of Ultraviolet Radiation to Control Acute Respiratory Disease', *Vestn Akad Med Nank SSSR*: 3; 37, 1975.

13 Levenson, S.M., et al., 'Nosocomial Infection: Prevention by Special Clean-Air, Ultraviolet Light, and Barrier Techniques', *Current Problems in Surgery*: XXIII no.7, 1986.

14 National Academy of Sciences National Research Council, Ad Hoc Committee. 'Postoperative Wound Infections: The Influence of Ultraviolet Irradiation of the Operating Room and of Various Other Factors', *Ann. Surg*: 160 (supp. 2); 1, 1964.

15 Hart, D., et al., 'Postoperative Wound Infections: A Further Report on Ultraviolet Irradiation', *Ann. Surg*: 167; 728, 1968.

16 Stevens, F.A., 'The Bactericidal Properties of Ultraviolet Irradiated Lipids of the Skin', *J. Exp Med*: 65; 121–126, 1937.

17 Crook, W. *The Yeast Connection*, Future Health Inc., Jackson, Tennessee.

18 Parrish, J.A., et al., 'Therapeutic Uses of Light', *Ann. New York Acad. Sci*: 453; 354–364, 1985.

Chapter ten

1 Perry, L.L., and Greens, M.I., 'Antigen Presentation by Epidermal Langerhans Cells: Loss of Function, Following

UV Irradiation in vivo', *Clin. Immunol. Immunopath*: 24; 204–219, 1982.

2 Granstein, R.D., et al., 'Epidermal Antigenpresenting Cells in Activation of Suppression'. *J. Immunol*: 132(2); 563–565, 1984.

3 Edelson, R.L., and Fink, J.M., 'The Immunologic Function of Skin', *Scientific American*: 252; 46–53, 1985.

4 Krenger, J., et al., 'Sleep Promoting Effects of Endogenous Pyrogen (Interleukin-1)', *Am. J. Physiol*: 246; R994, 1984.

5 Paul, W.E. (ed), *Fundamental Immunology*, Raven Press, New York, 1984.

6 Gahring, L., et al., 'Effect of Ultraviolet Radiation on Production of ETAF/Interleukin-1 in vivo and in vitro', *Proc Natl Acad Sci USA*: 81; 1198–1202, 1984.

7 Frick, G., 'Zur Wirkung der Ultravioletbestrahlung des Blutes auf das Blutbild, *Folia Haematol*: 101; 871–877, 1974.

8 Zabaluyera, A.P., 'General Immunological Reactivity of the Organism in Prophylactic UV Irradiation of Children in Northern Regions', *Vestn Akad Med Nank SSSR*: 3; 23, 1975.

9 Takno Fujita. et al., 'T-lymphocyte subsets in Osteoporosis', *J. Mineral Electr. Metab.*: 10; 375–378, 1984.

Chapter eleven

1 Black, H.S., and Rauschkolb, E.W., 'Effects of Light on Skin Lipid Metabolism', *J. Invest. Derm*: 56; 387–391, 1971.

2 Parrish, J.A., et al., 'Therapeutic Uses of Light', *Ann. New York Acad. Sci*: 453; 354–364, 1985.

3 Pathak, M.A., 'Activation of the Melanocyte System by Ultraviolet Radiation and Cell Transformation', *Ann. N.Y. Acad. Sci*: 453; 328–339, 1985.

4 Lever, W., and Schaumberg Lever, G., *Histopathology of the Skin*, 6th edition, Lippincott, Philadelphia, 1983.

5 Parrish, J.A., *J. Invest. Dermatol*: 77; 167–171, 1981.
6 Coyle, J.D., et al (eds), *Light, Chemical Change and Life'*, Open University Press, Milton Keynes, 1982.
7 Parrish, J.A., et al., *Arch. Dermatol*: 112; 1531–1534, 1976.
8 Kuiters, G.R., et al., 'Oral Phenylalanine Loading and Sunlight as Source of UVA Irradiation in Vitiligo on the Caribbean Island of Curacao', *J. Trop. Med. Hyg*: 89(3); 149–155, 1986.
9 Gschnait, F., et al., *Br. J. Dermatol*: 99; 293–295, 1978.
10 Rahn, O., *Invisible Radiations of Organisms*, Borntraeger, Berlin, 1936.
11 Dantsig, M., *Effect and Use of Ultraviolet Radiation (Ultrafioletovoye Izlucheniya)*, Meditsina Publishing House, Moscow, 1966.

Chapter twelve

1 Miley, G., 'The Ultraviolet Irradiation of AutoTransfused Human Blood: Studies in Oxygen Absorption Values', *Proc. Physiol. Soc, Philadelphia*, 17 April 1939.
2 Wassilieff, L.L., 'De l' influence de Travail Cerebral sur la Radiation Mitogenetique de sang', *Arch. Sciences Biol*: 35; 104, 1934.
3 Knott, E.K., 'Development of Ultraviolet Blood Irradiation', *Am. J. Surgery*: LXXVI, No 2; 165–171, 1948.
4 Levy, M., 'Der Einfluss Ultravioletter Strahlen auf die inneren Organe des Mans'. *Strahlentherapie*: 9; 618–623, 1919.
5 Dr. A. Rashid-Seyal, 'Blood Pressure and the Quality of Garments in the Young', 4th Ann. Internat. Symposium on Man and His Environment in Health and Disease. Dallas, 1986.
6 Allen, R.M., and Cureton, T.K., 'Effect of Ultraviolet Radiation on Physical Fitness', *Arch Phys med*: 26; 641–644, 1945.

7 Ohkawara, A., 'Glycogen Metabolism Following Ultraviolet Irradiation', *J. Invest Derm*: 59; 264–268, 1972.

8 Stewart, A., and Howard, J., 'Magnesium and Potassium Status of Women with Premenstrual Syndrome', 2nd European Congress on Magnesium, Stockholm, 1986.

9 Piesse, J.W., 'Nutrition Factors in the Premenstrual Syndrome', *Int. Nat. Clin. Rev:* Vol 4; 54–81, April 1984.

10 Pincussen, L., 'Effect of Ultraviolet and Visible Rays on Carbohydrate Metabolism', *Arch Phys Ther*: 18; 750–755, 1937.

11 Hollwich, F., 'The Effect of Natural and Artificial Light via the Eye on the Hormonal and Metabolic Balance of Animal and Man', *Ophthalmologica*: 180(4); 188–197, 1980.

12 Relkin, R. (ed), *The Pineal Gland*, Elsevier, New York, 1983.

13 Tanaka, Y., 'Effect of 1,25-Dihydroxyvitamin D3 on Insulin Secretion: Direct or Mediated', *Endocrinology*: 118(5); 1971–1974, 1986.

14 Durlach, J., and Klepping, J., 'Dietary Magnesium Intake Among Male Athletes in France', 2nd European Conference on Magnesium, Stockholm, 1986.

15 Darnall, L., 'The Pineal Gland and Ageing', *Complementary Medicine*: 2 no. 2; 47–51, 1986.

16 *Price's Textbook of the Practice of Medicine* (11th edition) Sir Ronald Bodley Scott (ed), Oxford University Press, 1973.

17 Ralph, C., 'Pineal Bodies and Thermoregulation', Relkin, R., (ed), *The Pineal Gland*, Elsevier, New York, 1983.

Chapter thirteen

1 Knutsson, A., et al., 'Increased Risk of Ischaemic Heart Disease in Shift Workers', *Lancet*: II; 89–92, 1986.

2 Tapp, W.N., 'Life Extension in Heart Disease: An Animal Model', *Lancet*: I; 238–239, 1986.

3 Rauschkolb, E.W., et al., 'Effect of Ultraviolet Light on Skin Cholesterol', *J. Invest Derm*: 49; 632–636, 1971.

4 Altschul, R., 'Ultraviolet Irradiation and Cholesterol Metabolism', *Arch Phys Med*: 36; 394–398, 1955.

5 Steenbock, H., 'Fat Soluble Vitamins: XIX', *J. Biol. Chem*: LXII(1); 209–217, 1924.

6 Altschul, R., and Hermann, I.H., 'Ultraviolet Irradiation and Cholesterol Metabolism', *Circulation*: 8; 438, 1953.

7 McDonagh, E.W., et al., 'The Clinical Change in Patients Treated with EDTA Chelation plus Multivitamin/Trace Mineral Supplementation', *J. Ortho Psych*: 14(1); 61–65, 1985.

8 McDonagh, E.W., et al., 'The Effect of Intravenous EDTA upon Blood Cholesterol in a Private Practice Environment', *J. Int. Acad. Prev. Med*: VII(1); 512, 1982.

9 Altschul, R., 'Inhibition of Experimental Cholesterol Arterosclerosis by Ultraviolet Irradiation', *New England Journal of Medicine*: 249; 96–100, 1953.

10 Seelig, M.S., 'Nutritional Status and Requirements of Magnesium', 2nd European Congress on Magnesium, Stockholm, 1986.

11 Metzler, D.E., *Biochemistry: The Chemical Reactions of Living Cells,* Academic Press, New York, 1977.

12 Rasmussen, H.S., et al., 'Magnesium and Acute Myocardial Infarction. Substituting Magnesium in Acute Myocardial: a Life Saver?' 2nd European Congress on Magnesium, Stockholm, 1986.

13 Lind, L., Wengle, B., and Ljunghall, S., 'Intermittent Hypercalcemia, Blood Pressure and Magnesium'. 2nd European Congress on Magnesium, Stockholm, 1986.

14 Abrahams, G.E., 'The Calcium Controversy', *J. Appl. Nutr*: 34,2; 69–73, 1982.

15 Lawson, D.E.M., in Diplock, A.T., (ed), *Fat Soluble Vitamins* Heinemann, London, 1985.

16 Miller, E.R., et al., 'Mineral Balance Studies with the Baby Pig', *J. Nutr*: 85; 255–259, 1965.

17 Meintzer, R., and Steenbock, H., 'Vitamin D and Magnesium Absorption', *J. Nutr*: 56; 285–294, 1955.

18 Seelig, M.S., 'Nutritional Status and Requirements of Magnesium', 2nd European Congress on Magnesium, Stockholm, 1986.

19 Petri, M., and Perry, R., 'Cellular and Plasma Magnesium in Diabetes', 2nd European Congress on Magnesium, Stockholm, 1986.

20 Laurens, H., 'The Physiologic Effects of Ultraviolet Radiation', *Journal of the American Medical Association*: 111; 2385–2392, 1939.

21 Johnson, J.R., et al., 'The Effect of Carbon Arc Radiation on Blood Pressure and Cardiac Output', *Am. J. Physiol*: 114; 594–602, 1935.

22 Allen, R.M., and Cureton, T.K., 'Effect of Ultraviolet Radiation on Physical Fitness', *Arch Phys Med*: 26; 641–644, 1945.

23 Mikhailov, V.A., 'Influence of Graduated Sunlight Baths on Patients with Coronary Atherosclerosis', *Soviet Med*: 29; 76–79, 1966.

24 Gabovich, R.D., et al., 'Effect of Ultraviolet Radiation on Tolerance of the Organism to Chemical Substances', *Vestn Akad Med Nauk SSSR*: 3; 26–28, 1975.

25 Dantsig, M., *Effect and Use of Ultraviolet Radiation, (Ultrafioletovoye Izlucheniya)*, Meditsina Publishing House, Moscow, 1966.

Chapter fourteen

1 Laurens, H., 'The Physiologic Effects of Ultraviolet Radiation', *Journal of the American Medical Association*: 111; 2385–2392, 1939.

2 Meintzer, R., and Steenbock, H., 'Vitamin D and Magnesium Absorption', *J. Nutr*: 56; 285–294, 1955.

3 Myerson, A., and Neustadt, R., 'Influence of Ultraviolet Irradiation upon Excretion of Sex Hormones In The Male', *Endocrinology*: 25; 7, 1939.

4 Aschoff, J., 'Annual Rhythms in Man', in Aschoff, J. (ed.), *Handbook of Behavioural Neurobiology*, Plenum Press, New York, 1981.

5 Williams, R., *Textbook of Endocrinology* 6th edition, W.B. Saunders, Philadelphia, 1981.

6 Marburg, O., 'Zur Kenntnis der Normalen und pathologischen Histologie der Zierbeldruse', *Arb Neur Inst, Wien*: 12; 217–279, 1909.

7 Waldhauser F., and Dietzel M., 'Daily and Annual Rhythms in Human Melatonin Secretion: Role in Puberty Control', *Ann. New York Acad. Sci*: 453; 205–214, 1985.

8 Waldhauser, F., et al., 'A possible role for Melatonin in Human Maturation', 3rd International Symposium on Psychoneuroendocrinology in Reproduction, Spoleto, Italy, 1985.

9 Hastings, M.H., et al., 'Annual Reproductive Rhythms in Mammals: Mechanisms of Light Synchronisation', *Ann. New York Acad. Sci*: 453: 182–204, 1985.

10 Cowgill, U.M., 'Season of Birth in Man. Contemporary situation with special reference to Europe and the Southern hemisphere', *Ecology*: 47; 614–623, 1966.

11 Watanabe, G.I., and Yoshida, S., 'Climatic Effect on Urinary Output of Neutral 17 ketosteroids', *J. Appl. Physiol*: 9; 456–460, 1956.

12 Rosenthal, N.E., et al., 'Seasonal Affective Disorder and Phototherapy', *Ann. New York Acad. Sci*: 435; 254–260, 1985.

Chapter fifteen

1 Lum on Hyperventilation.
2 Durlach, J., and Durlach, V. 'Idiopathic mitral valve Prolapse and Magnesium: State of the Art', 2nd European Congress on Magnesium. Stockholm, 1986.
3 Meintzer, R., and Steenbock, H., 'Vitamin D and Magnesium Absorption', *J. Nutr*: 56; 285–294, 1955.
4 Seelig, M.S., 'Nutritional Status and Requirements of Magnesium', 2nd European Congress on Magnesium, Stockholm, 1986.
5 Mikhailov, V.A., 'Influence of Graduated Sunlight Baths on Patients with Coronory Atherosclerosis', *Soviet Med*: 29; 76–79, 1966.
6 Ott, John, *Health and Light*, Pocket Books, New York, 1973.
7 Gabovich, R.D., et al., 'Effect of Ultraviolet Radiation on Tolerance of the Organism to Chemical Substances', *Vestn Akad Med Nauk SSSR*: 3; 2628, 1975.
8 Grant, Ellen, *The Bitter Pill*, Elm Tree Books, London 1985.
9 Mansfield, P., and Monro, J., *Chemical Children – How to Protect your Family from Harmful Pollutants*, Century Paperbacks, London, 1987.
10 Barnes, Broda O., *Hypothyroidism, The Unsuspected Illness*, Thomas Y. Crowell, New York, 1976.
11 William McKinley Jefferies, *Safe Uses of Cortisone*, Chas. C. Thomas, 1981.
12 Blackwell, H.R., 'Effects of Light Source Spectral Distribution upon Visual Functions', *Ann. New York Acad. Sci*: 453; 340–353, 1985.
13 Hedge, Alan, *Ill health among office workers in Ergonomies and health in modern offices*, Taylor & Francis, 1984.

Chapter sixteen

1 Luscher, M., *Farbenpsychologie*, Palette, Sandoz AG, Basel, 1959.

2 Revici, E., 'Research in Physiopathology as a basis of guided Chemotherapy with Special Application to Cancer', New York, 1961.

3 Klar, H., 'The Chi-Square Method in the Luscher Colour Test', *Medico*; 1, 1966.

4 Luscher, M., *Luscher Test*, Test-Verlag, Basel, 1948.

5 Ott, John, *Health and Light*, Pocket Books, New York, 1973.

6 Wohlfarth, H., 'The Effect of Colour-Psychodynamic Environmental Modification on Disciplinary Incidents in Elementary Schools Over One School Year: A Controlled Study', *Int. J. Biosoc. Res*: 1;44, 1984.

7 Wohlfarth, H., and Sam, C., *Effects of Colour/Light Changes on Severely Handicapped Children*, Planning & Research Division, Dept. of Education, Alberta, Canada, 1981.

8 Schauss, A., *Diet, Crime and Delinquency*, Parker House, Berkeley, 1980.

Index